After Prostate Cancer

After Prostate Cancer

*A What-Comes-Next Guide to a Safe
and Informed Recovery*

ARNOLD MELMAN, M.D.

ROSEMARY E. NEWNHAM

Published in the United States of America by Oxford University Press, Inc.,
198 Madison Avenue, New York, NY, 10016
United States of America

Oxford University Press, Inc., publishes works that further Oxford University's
objective of excellence in research, scholarship, and education

Oxford is a registered trade mark of Oxford University Press
in the UK and in certain other countries

Library of Congress Cataloging-in-Publication Data

Melman, Arnold.
  After prostate cancer : a what-comes-next guide to a safe and informed recovery / Arnold Melman and
Rosemary E. Newnham.
  p. cm.
  ISBN 978-0-19-539966-0 (acid-free paper)
  1. Prostate—Cancer—Patients—Rehabilitation. I. Newnham, Rosemary E. II. Title.
  RC280.P7M45   2011
  616.99'463—dc22

                                                                                      2010050193

ISBN 978-0-19-539966-0

1 3 5 7 9 10 8 6 4 2

Typeset in Chaparral-pro Regular
Printed on acid-free paper

Printed in the United States of America

CONTENTS

Prostate cancer is a very common yet very complex disease, one that has been heavily researched. As of this writing, over 90,000 peer-reviewed articles have been written on it. Even as an expert on prostate cancer who has devoted his career to the disease, it can be challenging for me to keep up with the myriad advances and understand all the nuances of the disease. Thankfully, Dr. Melman has taken the time to cull through the literature and share his wisdom with us on this complicated topic.

Current treatment of prostate cancer results in a cure for over 90% of patients. This means that many patients are living as prostate cancer survivors. In the United States alone, 200,000 men are diagnosed with prostate cancer each year, and there are now over 2.2 million American men who are prostate cancer survivors. Most books and references on prostate cancer focus on the first phase of the disease, the diagnosis and initial treatment decision. Issues related to living with the disease after initial treatment, including treatment side effects, recurrent cancer, and the impact of the disease on the patient's family, are often afterthoughts and do not receive the attention they deserve. Dr Melman has addressed these issues in the book, filling an important need for patients.

Dr. Melman is the right person to write this book and I believe it will serve as an authoritative and illuminating resource for patients and their loved ones for years to come. As the chairman of the urology department at the Montefiore Medical Center since 1986, he has trained over 70 residents, including myself. His inspiration and leadership have positively impacted all of our careers, and many of us have become leaders in urology as a result. He has written extensively about prostate cancer and erectile dysfunction, and is a world expert on the treatment of erectile dysfunction after prostatectomy.

During my residency, Dr. Melman was the first to teach me about prostate cancer, and he has been a valued mentor to me for over 15 years. Although he preferred the radical perineal prostatectomy, he encouraged me to try other approaches. To learn the open radical retropubic prostatectomy, I went on to complete a fellowship at Memorial Sloan-Kettering Cancer Center. Dr. Melman encouraged me to continue my education by learning laparoscopic prostatectomy in the only place it was being performed: France. During my fellowship there, the da Vinci robot was released, and I began to develop the robotic prostatectomy technique that I use to this day.

Since then, I have gone on to perform over 3,000 robotic prostatectomies. I still fondly remember Dr. Melman's lectures and teachings when I counsel and operate on my patients. Much of his wisdom and many of these lessons are included in this book. Having counseled thousands of men with prostate cancer, I know that it can often be difficult to answer all of their questions or communicate all the information they need in the short time that we have together. This book will be a useful adjunct to our conversation, a good resource that patients can use to help them cope with prostate cancer. I look forward to recommending it to all of my patients.

David B. Samadi, M.D.
Vice Chairman, Department of Urology
Chief, Division of Robotics and Minimally Invasive Surgery
The Mount Sinai Medical Center
New York, NY

Hope from hopelessness. That is the evolution I have seen in the diagnosis, treatment, and management of prostate cancer during the 40 years that I have been a urologist. When I began treating patients back in the 1970s, the majority of the men who walked through my door had an advanced stage of this disease—and many of them died from it—because there were no good ways to diagnose it early and few treatment options. Although prostate cancer is still the country's second leading cause of cancer death for men (after lung cancer), today's patients have a great advantage: the prostate-specific antigen (PSA) blood test allows us to diagnose the disease very early—all you have to do is get a yearly physical. That test, along with a range of modern treatment options, gives you a much greater chance of successful recovery—whether that means a complete cure or a chronic but manageable disease. And if you do experience complications from your treatment, there are a variety of remedies to fight these problems that simply weren't available 40 years ago. Over those 40 years, I have gained extensive experience guiding my patients through all the modern treatments as they battle prostate cancer, erectile dysfunction (ED), urinary incontinence (UI), and related problems.

By offering practical, well-founded medical information based on that experience, this book is intended to help the man with prostate cancer—and his wife or partner, family, and friends—deal with the issues that can arise through the course of the disease. Unfortunately, because prostate cancer is such a common disease, there is an overload of well-meaning but conflicting opinions about the "right" treatment by the "best" doctors: a one-size-fits-all approach that can leave an individual in a state of bewildered turmoil, hoping that the choices he makes are the right ones. We hope that this book can help you through these challenges by providing solid medical information as well as first-hand accounts from men who have themselves experienced different types of treatments and complications.

Specifically, our focus in this book is to help men who have been through prostate cancer treatment understand and negotiate post-treatment issues. The treatment could have been surgery, radiation, hormone treatment, watchful waiting, or a combination of these. No matter what the treatment, patients usually experience some challenges afterward; this book can help you handle those ups and downs and adjust to post-treatment life.

During my career as a urologist, I have had several areas of specialization, including prostate cancer and ED. For the past 10 years, I have been involved with the development of gene therapy for the treatment of ED. In 2000, I co-founded a company called Ion Channel Innovations, with the goal of proving the effectiveness of gene therapy. Chapter 11, devoted to future therapies, will describe that effort, as well as other promising ED and prostate cancer therapies in development.

My co-author, Rosemary Newnham, is a professional writer with a background in oral history and narrative medicine. For the past 6 years, she has facilitated creative writing workshops in hospitals, helping patients, staff, and family members process their experiences with cancer through the written word. Previously, she worked for many years with two projects that interviewed survivors of traumatic events: the Survivors of the Shoah Visual History Foundation in Los Angeles and the September 11th Narrative and Memory Project at Columbia University.

Together, we bring our expertise in caring for the whole patient to this book. We hope the information in the pages to come helps to ease your mind and your body as you work your way toward wellness.

ACKNOWLEDGMENTS

This book would not exist without the many prostate cancer patients who shared their thoughts and experiences with us and who allowed us to share them with our readers. In the course of our research, we spoke to many patients, who are quoted anonymously here, and one patient's wife, Leah Cohen. It takes a special kind of courage to open up about such private issues—thank you. We would also like to thank Leslie Schover, Ph.D., for her considerable contributions to the chapter on relationships.

We gratefully acknowledge our editor, Sarah Harrington, and the staff of Oxford University Press. Thank you for your patience.

ARNOLD MELMAN:

Foremost, I want to thank my wife Lois who, for nearly five decades, has uncomplainingly supported the demanding life of an academic clinician. Her understanding and encouragement allowed me to pursue yet another project that occupied innumerable nights and weekend hours that separated us from time together.

My interest and passion for perineal surgery were stimulated by my teachers at UCLA: Elmer Belt, a grand master of Urology in California, who developed the unique Belt approach to prostate; his nephew Willard Goodwin, first chairman at UCLA; Joe Kaufman; and Stan Brosman honed my skills to treat the afflictions of the prostate.

Kelvin P. Davies, my colleague at Einstein, has been gracious with his time and artistic talents to render numerous excellent drawings to make my anatomical descriptions more understandable.

Tom Pryor, an enthusiastic writer, made the connection to Rose Newnham possible that allowed us to work as a team to properly communicate the important issues to our intended audience.

Finally, my gratitude to the thousands of men and their partners whom I have cared for over the years who have shared with me their fears and concerns of not knowing what to do to face their prostate cancer. Those issues promulgated the idea to create this book to identify and discuss the issues in a down-to-earth but informative manner that could improve their quality of life.

ROSEMARY NEWNHAM:

Thank you to my writing colleague, Cris Beam, for putting me in touch with Arnold and to Arnold for being such a generous and interesting writing partner.

Heartfelt thanks to the members of the Narrative Medicine Workshop on the oncology unit at New York-Presbyterian Hospital for teaching me about cancer from every angle: patient, caretaker, and medical professional. I would especially like to recognize my beloved friend the late Pat Nixon, who proved that a life with cancer can still be a life of great joy.

My loving parents, Pat and Bob Newnham, a nurse and a scientist, put their considerable skills and their generous hearts into making the world a better place: I endeavor to live up to their example. My father died during the writing of this book, and I am grateful that my life situation allowed me to love and care for him to the end and now to provide support for my mother as well. Thank you to my brother Randy, my extended family, and my friends for the love and laughter that sustain me. Loving gratitude to my husband Patrick for his big heart, big brain, and big bowls of ice cream, as well as his technical expertise in footnotes and foot rubs. (Our book is next, honey!) Finally, there's an extra wonderful reason why this book went to press a little later than planned: his name is Henry Everest and he was born in January 2010. May he know a long, happy life full of good love and good health.

After Prostate Cancer

1

The Basics of the Prostate and Prostate Cancer

About 2 million men in the United States today are living with prostate cancer or the after-effects of the disease. Prostate cancer affects one in six men in this country: almost 218,000 men were diagnosed with it in 2010.[1] Clearly, it is a health problem that many men have to face and make decisions about—before, during, and after treatment. It is our hope that this book can lessen the anxiety involved with these decisions and help you make the best choices for your improved health and well-being. Although it may be unpleasant to read about some of the repercussions of this illness, we hope that the more you know, the more empowered you will feel to make good decisions in your current and future healthcare—so let's start with the basics.

We want to begin by giving some fundamental information about the prostate and prostate cancer as well as the various treatment options. The basic overview of the first two chapters will set the scene for a fuller discussion of the side effects involved with treatment. Chapters 3 through 6 will cover the two most common side effects—erectile dysfunction and urinary incontinence—and their treatment. Less common side effects are discussed in Chapter 7, and treatment for advanced disease is discussed in Chapter 8. Chapter 9 deals with the psychological aspects of recovery and Chapter 10 with associated relationship issues. In the final chapter, we will discuss research and testing being done now on future treatments for prostate cancer and its complications.

THE PROSTATE GLAND AND ITS FUNCTION

The prostate gland in an adult male is about the size of a small kiwi fruit and is located around the urethra (the tube through which men urinate and ejaculate), where the urethra and the bladder meet. The prostate gland is composed of four main zones—one of which, the transition zone, is a central area that becomes enlarged when a man develops benign prostate disease (*see* page 5). As shown in Figure 1.1, the front, or apex, of the prostate gland faces the base of the penis. The back side of the gland sits immediately in front of the rectum and therefore can be felt during rectal examination by your physician. This back part of the prostate is where 80% of all prostate cancers begin to grow, so as uncomfortable as rectal exams are, they are very useful in catching cancer early.

The main function of the prostate gland is to produce most of the fluid part of male ejaculate. Only 1% of ejaculate is actually sperm—the rest is liquid that keeps the sperm alive and helps it achieve its object of uniting with the female egg. It can be confusing: *Glands* are small groups of cells that produce secretions (such as insulin or hormones) that help the body do a specific job; but the prostate itself is also called a *gland*; in this case, the term means an organ that produces a secretion. In the prostate, the product manufactured by the glands is fluid that helps keep sperm alive after ejaculation. So the prostate gland has a

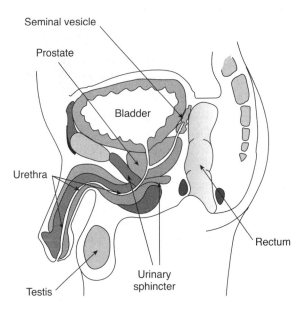

Figure 1.1 A view of the male pelvis with the relationships of the organs to one another from the side. (Courtesy of Kelvin Davies, Ph.D.)

specific function designed to help keep our species alive through reproduction. It also means that once men are finished with their reproductive years, they no longer need to have a prostate gland.

As you can see in Figure 1.1, the urethra runs through the middle of the prostate, and that section of the urethra is called the prostatic urethra. Think of the urethra as a highway that runs from the bladder out to the tip of the penis. Urine takes the expressway from the bladder, straight through the prostate, and out the penis. When a man ejaculates, the seminal vesicles and the ejaculatory ducts under the bladder contract, pushing sperm into the prostate, where it mixes with the liquid prostate secretions. At the moment of orgasm, the final product jumps onto an "on ramp" from the prostate onto the prostatic urethra and out the tip of the penis.

BENIGN PROSTATE DISEASE

It is common for the prostate to grow with age, which can partially block the urethra and make it harder to urinate. The most common cause of prostate enlargement is a non-cancerous condition called benign prostatic hyperplasia (BPH). More than half of men in their 60s have symptoms of BPH, and 90% of men have them by the time they reach their 70s and 80s. BPH is an increase in the number of glands that immediately surround the urethra, in the "transition zone" of the prostate. As the transition zone grows bigger, it begins to squash the prostatic urethra, making it narrower. As a result, you might notice that it takes longer to begin the stream, that the force of the stream is less (you can no longer write your name in the snow), or you might feel that you are not able to empty your bladder and consequently must urinate again just a few minutes later. Other symptoms can include feeling an urgency to urinate, waking up many times during the night to go to the bathroom, or dribbling urine into your shorts after you finish urinating. Figure 1.2 shows an enlarged prostate.

If you have these symptoms, there are several important reasons to get them checked out by your doctor. First, there are treatments for BPH that can you make you more comfortable by easing your symptoms. And second, the same symptoms can also arise as a result of the urethra being squeezed by a tumor.

PROSTATE CANCER

Prostate cancer is much less common then BPH, although it is a disease that also often comes with age—more than 80% of prostate cancers are diagnosed in men older than 65 years. Unlike BPH, which affects 50% to 90% of men,

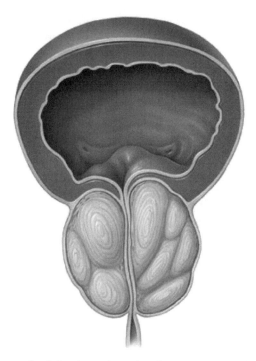

Figure 1.2 A prostate gland that has enlarged and is compressing the urethra passing through the center of the gland. The enlarged prostate also obstructs outflow of urine from the bladder.
(Courtesy of American Medical Systems, Minnetonka, Minnesota;
www.americanmedicalsystems.com.)

prostate cancer carries a 20% or less risk (Caucasian men have a 17% chance of being diagnosed with prostate cancer during their lifetime, and African-American men have a 20% chance). As mentioned above, rapidly fatal cases of prostate cancer have become much more rare and have reached new lows in the last several years because of improved modes of diagnosis and treatment. The 5-year survival rate (a typical statistic used to measure cancer outcomes) is nearly 100%. Of course, most patients live much longer, continuing happy and productive lives. Others—usually those whose cancer was already advanced at diagnosis—may not have as many years but should still do everything they can to maximize their health to feel as good as they can for as long as they can. The fact that men do still die of this disease should serve as a strong motivation for all men to get annual prostate exams so any potential cancer can be defeated before it spreads.

The difference between BPH and prostate cancer is that with cancer, the glands cells simply do not know when to stop growing—they grow and reproduce in an unlimited and uncontrollable manner. The vast majority of cases are diagnosed as localized cancer, which means that the cancer growth stays confined within the prostate gland. In some cases, the cancer does spread outside of the prostate to other organs and parts of the body. The spread of cancer cells outside the area of origin is called metastasis (*see* Chapter 8 for a discussion of metastasized cancers and their treatment). The effects of those metastasized cells in parts of the body where they do not belong causes the most problems and the most prostate cancer deaths. This explains why doctors are so focused on catching and treating this cancer early, before it has a chance to spread.

As with BPH, the symptoms of prostate cancer include difficulty urinating or decreased strength of the urine stream. Often, however, men with early stage prostate cancer have no symptoms at all and are discovered only through a physical exam or PSA test. Prostate cancer can have other symptoms, however, especially if it is an advanced case: pain in your abdomen, pain in your back or hip bones, pain during urination, or even blood in the urine or semen.

DIAGNOSING PROSTATE CANCER

Men with prostate cancer often have no symptoms at all: the first sign is a call from their doctor's office to discuss their test results, or a worried look on their doctor's face after a physical. We cannot emphasize enough that every man should have an annual physical exam that includes a digital rectal exam and a PSA blood test (*see* pages 8–12 for a discussion of PSA tests and who should get them). These exams are two very effective tools doctors use to find prostate cancer. If the results of either of these tests are unexpected, then a doctor will often take further steps, such as more advanced testing or a biopsy of the prostate, to make a definitive diagnosis.

Digital Rectal Exam

Although few people object to having their heart or abdomen examined, many men are reluctant to have a digital rectal examination (DRE). Some patients have told me in retrospect that they felt embarrassed (or worse) by the exam, even when it was performed in a routine, rapid, and entirely painless manner. For many patients, it is the most uncomfortable (both physically and mentally) part of their annual physical. Believe it or not, it is not the doctor's favorite moment either, but it is essential in that it yields information about your prostate that cannot be gained any other way. (A DRE can also be done for other reasons, such as to check for bleeding in the GI tract or to "harvest" a stool sample.)

In terms of the prostate, the rectal exam allows the physician to directly palpate an organ that may have a cancer in it, feeling around for any unusual lumps or textures. A healthy prostate will feel similar to the flexed muscle at the base of your thumb. If the doctor feels something that seems unusual, hard or irregular, or changed since the last exam, he will consider a biopsy, depending on the seriousness of the lump and the results of your PSA test. The presence of a lump does not always mean that cancer is present. The lump could be a small area of benign enlargement, a stone in the meat of the prostate, or scar tissue.

Prostate-Specific Antigen Test

PSA stands for *prostate-specific antigen*, an enzyme manufactured by prostate cells. The function of PSA is to liquefy semen to allow sperm greater mobility on their pilgrimage to the female's egg. Like many other substances made in the body's cells, a small proportion of PSA leaks into the bloodstream and can be measured by a blood test. In a man with or without cancer, the presence of PSA in the bloodstream is harmless and of no concern whatsoever. In a man with prostate cancer, the amount of PSA is very important because it is an indication of prostate cell activity: when cells start multiplying in the prostate like crazy (like they do when they are cancerous), then activity goes up, and in general so does the level of PSA.

Unlike many other blood tests, there is no standard baseline score for the PSA test; the normal amount of PSA in a man's blood depends on the size and "leakiness" of his prostate. Two men could have the same number: it could be normal for one man and be a sign of prostate cancer for the other. However, there are scores that could signal changes. For example, if you have a very high PSA number or an increase of 0.75 or more in a year, this means there has been a sudden jump in prostate activity, which could indicate an inflammation or possibly cancer. Most doctors would recommend that further tests be done to determine what is going on. Most often a doctor would start with a thorough clinical exam (including a rectal exam) and other PSA tests for free PSA and PSA velocity and density before suggesting a biopsy to search for cancer.

The discovery of using a PSA blood test to help diagnose prostate cancer is one of the great advances in medicine, and it happened only about 30 years ago. Scientists isolated PSA in 1980, and by 1986 the first commercial PSA blood test was released. Before this test was discovered, there was no reasonable way to make the diagnosis of early prostate cancer, and because prostate cancer has few symptoms until the disease is advanced, about half of the men had metastatic prostate cancer by the time of diagnosis. Today, because of PSA testing, there has been a 40% reduction in prostate cancer deaths since the 1990s, and it is rare for a man to arrive at the doctor with obvious metastatic disease.

WHAT YOUR PROSTATE-SPECIFIC ANTIGEN SCORE MEANS (AND DOESN'T MEAN)

There is no specific normal number for PSA because the size of prostate and "leakiness" of PSA into the bloodstream are different for everyone, making it difficult to ascertain what is normal or abnormal for any given man. With that said, researchers have studied large numbers of men and their PSA values and have established cut-off levels to better separate men who have infections or BPH from those who have prostate cancer. In addition to BPH, some other non-cancerous diseases can cause elevation of the PSA, including prostate infection or inflammation, recent ejaculation, and prostatic infarct (the rapid increase and death of a small area of the prostate that outgrows its blood supply).

Some medications can falsely lower the PSA and mask a high number. Remember to tell your doctor if you are taking a drug for any prostate symptoms. Some prescription medications (finasteride [Proscar], dutasteride [Avodart]) and over the counter supplements that contain the natural product Saw Palmetto can lower the blood PSA by as much as 50%.

PSA is reported as nanograms (ng) per milliliter (mL) in the blood. A nanogram is a billionth of a gram, and there are 28.35 g in 1 ounce of a liquid. That means that the actual amount of PSA in the blood is miniscule and is measurable only because laboratory technology has advanced so much in the past few decades.

The newest research suggests that the previously used cut-off value of 4.0 ng/mL as abnormal should be lowered to 2.5 or 3.0, because in a recent sizable study, prostate cancer was diagnosed in 15% of men with a PSA at or below 4.0 ng/mL. What makes those numbers even more significant is that 15% of *those* men had aggressive cancers. Some have suggested the use of age-specific PSA reference ranges. However, their use may lead to missing as many as 20% of cancer diagnoses in men in their 60s and 60% for men in their 70s.[2]

If one uses total PSA alone to decide who to biopsy for prostate cancer, then the 25% to 35% of the men biopsied will have a positive diagnosis, but that means that as many as 75% do not have prostate cancer and will have had an unnecessary biopsy.[3] To avoid the pain and expense of a biopsy, urologists rely on other means to try to make the early and correct diagnosis of prostate cancer, including free versus total PSA.

> "The PSA was just a test. You don't think it's something that will happen to you. Sometimes you wake up and think it's all a bad dream."
>
> —Reggie M.

FREE PROSTATE-SPECIFIC ANTIGEN AS AN INDICATOR FOR PROSTATE CANCER

The PSA in the bloodstream in is in two forms: attached to a protein molecule (total PSA) or not attached to a protein (free PSA). The common PSA blood test numbers usually refer to total PSA only. When prostate cancer cells release PSA into the bloodstream, it is more likely to stick to protein molecules than PSA released by BPH cells. That means that if a person has prostate cancer, his *free* PSA levels are likely to be lower than a person with BPH. The lower the free PSA, the more likely a cancer will be found. Thus, the free PSA has become another index of when to do the biopsy. If the urologist does biopsies on the results of total PSA alone, then he will do more unnecessary biopsies.

Free PSA is usually calculated as a percent of the total PSA. For example, if your free PSA is 20%, this would mean that 20% of the PSA in your bloodstream is free, or unattached, PSA. You want to see a higher number here because *the more free PSA, the less likely it is cancer*. I favor using a free PSA of 16% or lower as an indication for when to do the biopsy. Table 1.1 below details the approximate probability of having prostate cancer for a range of free PSA percentiles is as follows:[4]

Table 1.1. FREE PSA

% Free PSA (if total PSA = 4–10 ng/mL)	Probability of prostate cancer
25% or higher	8%
20–25%	16%
15–20%	20%
10–15%	28%
0–10%	56%*

*It is significant that even when the free PSA is at its lowest, the probability of *not* having a cancer is still 44%.

PROSTATE-SPECIFIC ANTIGEN DENSITY AND VELOCITY AS INDICATORS OF PROSTATE CANCER

Another helpful predictor is PSA density, which is the ratio of the total PSA to the size of the prostate. For example, a man with a PSA of 10 ng/mL and a prostate gland measured at 100 g has a PSA density of 10/100, or 0.1. Benign tissue secretes more PSA per gram then cancerous tissue, so it is natural for a man with a large prostate to have a higher PSA. When a man with a smaller prostate has a very high PSA, it can be a red flag. Most doctors use a ratio of 0.16 as a cut-off for deciding when to do a biopsy. Therefore, two men could have the same total PSA number (4 ng/mL), but the man with a 25-g prostate (density 0.16) might get a biopsy, whereas the man with a 50-g prostate (density 4/50 or 0.08) would not. This number would be determined by a transrectal ultrasound, the only way to determine the size of the prostate.

PSA velocity means the change in PSA level over a year. As we age, our prostates tend to grow, so it is normal to have some elevation of PSA from year to year, but the current information suggests that if the PSA increases more than 0.35 ng/mL in a year, then a biopsy should be performed. As covered above, a jump in PSA usually reflects a jump in prostate gland activity, which could mean that an inflammation or cancer is present.

RECOMMENDATIONS FOR PROSTATE-SPECIFIC ANTIGEN TESTS

These figures highlight the importance of annual or biannual PSA tests (preferably processed by the same laboratory to limit any lab-to-lab variation in results) in diagnosing prostate cancer. In our current insurance-based health system, where costs are always a top concern, there is some controversy about when, how often, and for whom PSA tests should be obtained. The controversy exists because both cancerous and normal cells make PSA, and therefore a high PSA level may be found in men without cancer.

There are many conflicting reports about testing PSA in the media today. They revolve around a few major issues, especially:

1. The cost of the test to the government and insurance companies;
2. The issue of whether the tests really do help save lives;
3. Debate about at what ages testing should begin and stop.

Because so many sincere and knowledgeable medical professionals disagree, it makes the average Joe's decision whether to obtain a routine PSA blood test even harder. My own philosophy is that since the introduction of PSA testing, prostate cancers have been caught earlier and therefore there has been a very substantial decrease in the death rate from prostate cancer (40% according to the American Cancer Society). Even if the man may eventually die from this disease, he can live longer with it because he has received treatment to prolong his life. To my mind, that is an advance that is worth every penny, and I believe that you as an individual should demand to have a PSA test done regularly by your healthcare provider.

The latest recommendations by the American Urological Association and the National Comprehensive Cancer Network is to offer both a yearly PSA test and a digital rectal exam (to try to find small tumors on the rectal side of the prostate that are not secreting large amounts of PSA) from *at least* ages 50 to 75 years. Medicare and the U.S. Food and Drug Administration (FDA) have also approved the use of the PSA test and the DRE over the age of 50. Men with a family history of prostate cancer (father, brother, cousin, uncle) and African-American men (because they have the highest incidence of prostate cancer in the United States) should begin at age 40 years. The age at which you stop having an annual test depends on your overall health and family history. If you are 75, in good health, and still taking care of your 95-year-old mother, then you have a similar chance to live to a very ripe old age and should continue the testing.

A PATIENT'S STORY: DIAGNOSIS AS A RESULT OF PROSTATE-SPECIFIC ANTIGEN

In his mid-50s, Richard D. had a job that required an annual physical but did not include a PSA test. A few months after his physical, he went to a urologist for a minor health problem and while he was there got his PSA tested, mainly because he didn't know his score and thought it was probably time to find out. His score came back at 5.4, high enough that his doctor scheduled a biopsy for the next week, commenting: "You're much too young to have a score that high." Very soon after his biopsy, Richard got a call from the urologist, who said, "I want you to come in tomorrow with your wife." At that moment, Richard knew, "You're telling me I've got cancer." "Yup," said his doctor. Not just a small cancer, either, but one that had taken over almost his whole prostate. The urologist estimated in about three more months it would have spread to the bone. Richard decided, "If it's bad, let's get it out and get on with my life." He had a prostatectomy and now, almost 20 years and several grandchildren later, is still cancer-free.

The Next Step: Biopsy

Once your physician has determined that you need a biopsy, you will make an appointment for a transrectal biopsy, the only way to make the diagnosis of prostate cancer. Although this doesn't sound like much fun, today's method of doing prostate biopsies is one of the great advances (along with PSA testing) in making an early diagnosis of prostate cancer. Years ago, a prostate biopsy was a long and painful surgical experience. Today, the transrectal ultrasound allows a fast, (fairly) painless, and very thorough examination of the prostate by the doctor in an outpatient setting. The probe the doctor inserts into the rectum is about the thickness of a cigar; the test lasts about 2 minutes and feels the same as a rectal examination. The ultrasound waves measure the size and shape of the prostate and can also show any abnormal lesions on the prostate.

Your doctor will decide in advance to just do a simple ultrasound or to do an ultrasound and a biopsy. To biopsy the prostate, a needle is passed through the ultrasound probe via a device known as the Biopty gun. Thanks to local anesthesia and the invention of the Biopty gun, the biopsy can be done painlessly and quickly—almost always less than 5 minutes. My patients tell me that the worst part of the test is the popping noise made by the "gun" when it fires the needle into the prostate to remove the tissue.

During a biopsy, most urologists remove 12 tiny pieces of the prostate from different areas on each side of the gland, which are sent to a pathology lab for analysis. Because the needle passes through the rectum to reach the prostate, the primary risk of the procedure is infection. An antibiotic must be given before the procedure in order to prevent that from happening, but a small percentage of men get fever and chills from infection and may need further care even when they take the antibiotic first. Nevertheless, the advantage of early cancer diagnosis of cancer far outweighs the risk of infection.

Remember that a negative biopsy does not necessarily mean that there is not cancer present. The needles are small and take small representative samples of the prostate. If a cancer is present but still very small, the biopsy needle may miss the cancerous area. Follow-up PSA tests after a few months are still necessary–especially if there are potentially questionable areas on the biopsy specimen.

STAGING THE PROSTATE CANCER

You will feel more comfortable about the decisions you are making before, during, and after your treatment if you are equipped with good information when communicating with your medical team. One of the most important aspects of your situation to learn about is the stage of your cancer at diagnosis. The "stages" of cancer are used by physicians to describe the extent of the cancer at a specific time. It is from the presumed stage—the cancer's size, location, and aggressiveness—that all other treatment decisions will flow. (We say "presumed" because occasionally additional discoveries made during treatment cause a doctor to revise the stage at a later time; *see* page 127 for more information.)

The most commonly used system for staging cancers is the TMN system. The "T" or Tumor describes the size and location of the cancer. Specifically for prostate cancer staging, T1 is small and confined to the prostate; T2 cancer is larger and can involve one or both lobes of the prostate but it remains confined to the gland; T3 cancer extends outside the gland into local tissues; and T4 is metastatic cancer that has spread to more distant regions or organs. If the cancer has spread, your doctor may assign additional staging using "M"s or "N"s. The "M" stands for metastasis to other organs and "N" for cancer spread to one or more lymph nodes.

To determine the stage of your cancer, the doctors need to know the location, amount, and aggressiveness of your cancer. Additional tests are required to answer these questions, but hopefully they will be quick and painless for you. Doctors use four main procedures to help gage those factors: scans, Gleason's Score, clinical exam, and PSA.

Scans

Scans, or imaging procedures, are needed to help determine location of the tumor(s). There are three or four scans used in prostate cancer staging. The first, a transrectal ultrasound, is part of the biopsy procedure. An ultrasound wand is placed into the rectum, an ideal location to map the size of the patient's prostate and give direction to the urologist doing the biopsy. Unfortunately this procedure is rarely helpful in seeing the actual cancer cells.

Next, you may be sent for a computed tomography (CT) scan of the pelvic area. This scan can help your doctor see if any of the lymph nodes in the area are enlarged—they have to be significantly bigger, more than half an inch in size, to be seen on this scan.

An endorectal magnetic resonance imaging (MRI) is a modified MRI test in which a large probe is placed in the rectum for about 45 minutes. This is not comfortable, but it does allow for excellent imaging of the prostate. Various permutations of this test are called dynamic contrast MRI, MR spectroscopy, and diffusion-weighted MR imaging. In a recent study, when all three of these tests were performed, they were nearly 100% accurate for identifying the cancer in and around the prostate. By themselves, they were accurate about 60% of the time.[5] Most doctors, however, will not put patients through every kind of MRI test. In most cases, a less than 100% accuracy rate is sufficient for treatment. Furthermore, the tests are expensive, may not be covered by insurance, and the equipment may not be available in your area.

If a patient has a very high PSA (more than 20 ng/mL) and Gleason's grade (8–10), or bone pain, it is likely that the prostate cancer has spread beyond the prostate itself (a Stage 3, non-localized cancer). In these cases, the man will be tested for bone metastases with a nuclear medicine test called a bone scan. In that test, the patient is injected intravenously with a radioactive material that is drawn to the bones. A few hours later, the patient lays on a table that measures radiation around the body. In the event of areas of increased bone activity (such as bone cancer or an infection), the radiation is more active and shows up brightly on the scan. If there are signs of bone activity, then the results of the scan will be confirmed with MRI and/or biopsy before a definite diagnosis is made.

The Gleason's Score

After your biopsy is completed, your tissue samples are sent to a pathology lab, where they are placed on microscope slides and studied by a pathologist. A pathologist is an MD who studies diseases by examining minute changes in the body's fluids and tissues—they are the living patients' equivalent of the forensic pathologists you see on TV cop shows who find the killer's DNA from a single strand of hair left at the crime scene.

Dr. Donald Gleason was a pathologist in Minneapolis Veteran's Association Medical Center in the 1960s and 1970s. Studying microscope slides of prostate cancer cells all day long, Gleason realized that the pattern of cancerous cells he saw on the slides could help predict the likelihood that the tumor would spread. He gave the most common pattern observable on a given slide a score of 1 to 5 (1 being closely packed, more "normal"-looking cell pattern and more benign cancer; 5 being very diffuse, irregular cell patterns). He then gave the second most common pattern he saw on the same slide another score of 1 to 5. Adding together the numbers associated with the first and second most common cell patterns gave a final score ranging from 2 to 10. Often, however, the score is given in the form of $x + y$ (x being the first most common pattern, y the second); for example, a score of $3 + 4$ or $4 + 3$ would both give a final score of 7 but could mean different things in terms of your cancer's aggressiveness. Cancers with total scores between 2 and 6 are less likely to escape the prostate, scores of 8 to 10 are much more likely to spread (*see* Table 1.2 below). Your physician will use

Table 1.2. GLEASON'S SCORE

Gleason's score	Cancer aggressiveness	Prognosis
3 + 3 (total of 6 or less)	Low-grade	Favorable
3 + 4 / 3 + 5	Mostly low-grade with some high	Reasonable
4 + 3 / 5 + 3	Mostly high-grade with some low	Reasonable
4 + 4 / 4 + 5 / 5 + 4 / 5 + 5	Tumor all high-grade	Cancer more likely to spread

the Gleason's score of your biopsied cancer cells to help determine the aggressiveness of your prostate cancer. (*See* Table 2.1 on page 20 for more details.)

Dr. Gleason's scale, patented in 1974, provided an accepted standard for evaluating prostate cancers. Previous to that time, every pathology department developed their own standards, leading to considerable confusion (especially if a patient moved from one hospital to another for treatment) and impeding research into new treatments.

Clinical Exam

The main way that location and extent of a cancer is determined by physical examination is through a DRE, done in the doctor's office (*see* page 7 for a basic description). Although DRE is a tool for diagnosis, it is also relied upon to help stage prostate cancer, because if there is a lump or nodule, the doctor can often feel where the tumors are and how big they are through a DRE. Sometimes the doctor can accurately stage a tumor by the DRE; other times the information gained through the DRE is combined and cross-referenced with information gained from scans about size and location of the cancer.

In today's world, because of the well-publicized need for PSA tests and rectal examinations, most prostate cancers fall into the T1 category because the cancer does not have an opportunity to grow before being discovered. In my experience it is the men who are afraid of the possible result, suspicious of the test, or refuse to have the testing that have the T2 or higher tumors and therefore

Table 1.3. The Stages of Prostate Cancer as noted through DRE

T1: normal digital rectal examination

T1a: less than 5% of prostate (can only be discovered accidentally when treating for another medical issues, such as an operation for BPH)

T1b: more than 5% of prostate (but still can only be discovered accidentally)

T1c: very small amount but found during a biopsy done because of an elevated PSA

T2: a nodule or hardness that is still confined to the prostate

T2a: a nodule or hardness involving less than one-half of one side of the prostate

T2b: nodule involving more the one-half of one side of the prostate

T2c: nodule involving both sides of the prostate

T3: tumor extends outside the prostate

T3a: tumor spread outside the capsule of the prostate on one or both sides (but not yet spread into any other organ)

T3b: tumor spread to the seminal vesicles

T4: evidence that the tumor has extended or spread into other organs such as the rectum or bladder a higher chance of dying from the disease. If a patient does have a meta-stasized cancer (stage 3 or 4), his tumor's stage classification would also carry an "M" for metastasis to other organs and perhaps even an "N" to signal cancer is also in lymph nodes. These other letters would also have a number to grade the severity of the cancer—for example, T3M1N2.

TREATMENT GOAL

When doctors diagnose cancer in a patient, they decide on the goals of the treatment and that goal will inform all future decisions. In most cases, the goal is either to cure the cancer or to suppress and control its growth. If you've gone through treatment already but are unsure what the treatment goals were in your case, or how aggressive your cancer was/is, ask your doctor now.

Most of the treatments that we will describe in the next chapter are for local-ized prostate cancer—that is, cancer that is confined to the prostate gland. Usually the intent of the treatment offered for localized cancer will be to cure the cancer. If the tumor has already spread to other organs (i.e., metastasized) at the time of diagnosis, then the treatment offered will aim to suppress or con-trol the cancer's growth, not to cure it. The hope is to convert cancer into a chronic disease that can be controlled with careful treatment. Think of diseases like high blood pressure, heart disease, or diabetes—with vigilance and proper medical care, people with these illnesses can live happy and productive (although changed) lives for a long time.

Once your medical team has diagnosed your cancer and determined its stage, it is time to decide what your treatment goals are and which treatment to pursue.

2

Prostate Cancer Treatments

CHOOSING A TREATMENT FOR LOCALIZED DISEASE

In most cases, the goal for treating localized disease is to cure the cancer, whether by cutting it out (surgery), burning it out (radiation), cooking or freezing it (*see* Chapter 11 for information on HIFU and cryotherapy), starving it (hormone suppression therapy; Chapter 8) or some combination of these. The hoped-for outcome is no more cancer and many more years of productive living. You will note that the goal is not to return you to your pre-cancer life. Of course, doctors and patients alike hope that the patient will feel every bit as healthy after treatment as before the cancer diagnosis, but in almost every case, there are at least some changes in the body as a result of the cancer and/or its treatment. Any doctor who guarantees that you will be "right back to normal" after treatment is overstating the case. Doctors should say that you will have a new "normal", hopefully one very similar to your pre-cancer life, but not necessarily. The doctor's primary goal is always to get rid of the cancer in order to save your life.

No matter which treatment option you choose, a great deal of your future quality of life is determined by the cards you were dealt when your diagnosis was made, such as the size and aggressiveness of your cancer. The good news is that the prostate-specific antigen (PSA) test now allows the diagnosis of prostate cancer at a much earlier stage and that, along with a range of modern, patient-friendlier treatment options, gives a much greater chance of successful recovery either as a complete cure of the cancer or as a chronic, but manageable, disease over many years.

What will your outcome be? Statistics can give you summaries of various treatment outcomes, based on what happened to others under similar circumstances. (*See* page 44 at the end of this chapter for a table summarizing some of the current literature results.) However, for any one individual, there is no current scientific tool to accurately predict the way a particular cancer will grow, no matter what the appearance of the cancer under the pathologist's microscope. Some cancers that look perfectly benign grow rapidly and quickly become unresponsive to treatment, whereas other tumors that appear more aggressive may not. My advice to my patients is to be as aggressive in treatment as possible to cure a potentially curable cancer. Of course, that advice must be realistically modified by the person's age, overall health, social situation, and willingness and ability to pursue the best opportunity for cure.

For example, I once was asked to give a second opinion for a man who had been diagnosed with early stage, localized prostate cancer. He was 54 years old and in perfect health. Most urologists, myself included, would have recommended that he have a radical prostatectomy (surgery) for his best chance of cure. However, he had a unique problem in that he was the sole caregiver for two young children and could not take even the slightest chance that any prolonged illness or death would occur with surgery, as there was no one else to care for his children. He elected to have external beam radiation therapy (EBRT) as his therapy, and I agreed with his choice even though I thought it a compromise for his *best* chances of long-term cure.

PROSTATE CANCER AGGRESSIVENESS AND RELATED CARE OPTIONS

Your treatment options are, to a degree, dictated by the stage of your cancer at diagnosis, but for most people, there is still some choice involved with their treatment decision. Prostate cancer aggressiveness risk scores and care options for early stage localized prostate cancer have been compiled by the National Comprehensive Cancer Network Guidelines and are summarized in Table 2.1.[1]

Let's take a look at the main types of treatment for localized prostate cancer: surgery, watchful waiting, radiation, and combination therapy.

Table 2.1. EARLY STAGE PROSTATE CANCER ONLY
(LOCALIZED TO PROSTATE GLAND)

Aggressiveness category	Gleason's score (total)	Clinical stage*	PSA	Options
Low risk of spreading beyond the prostate	6 or less	T1 or T2a	< 10	Watchful waiting, surgery, brachytherapy, or external beam radiation
Intermediate risk of spreading	6 or greater	T1, T2a or b	10–20 or ≤ 20	Surgery, brachytherapy, or external beam radiation with ADT**
High risk of spreading	7 or greater	T1,T2a,b or c	> 20 or any PSA	Surgery or external beam radiation with ADT

* DRE scores greater than T2 are cancers that have already spread outside the prostate. See Chapter 8 for more on treatment for advanced disease.
** ADT = androgen suppression therapy, or hormone therapy

SURGICAL PROSTATE CANCER TREATMENTS

Surgery for prostate cancer is designed to cure the cancer by removing the entire prostate gland, with all of its contained cancer cells, and the immediate surrounding tissues into which the cancer cells may have spread. For most men, deciding to have surgery "down there" is a difficult choice to make—but a lot of men do make that decision. In 2009, almost 200,000 men were diagnosed with prostate cancer in the United States, and about half were treated with surgery. Removal of the prostate gland—a procedure called a prostatectomy—can offer patients the best chance to permanently cure their cancer. During a prostatectomy, the entire prostate and the adjacent organs, the seminal vesicles, are removed. Surgical technique has improved so dramatically that it has become a routine operation with a very low chance of serious operative complications or death. In all cases of prostate surgery, patients are given anesthesia to ensure they feel no pain during the operation, and the recovery—particularly if the newer methods are used—is also relatively painless.

There are several methods of performing a radical prostatectomy. The word "radical" is used to describe cancer surgery in which more than just the affected organ is removed—in this case, it refers to the adjacent seminal vesicles and ejaculatory ducts that are removed along with the prostate gland. The seminal vesicles store fluid and the ejaculatory ducts store ejaculatory fluid and sperm (*see* Figure 5.1). These two glands are removed because they are a functional component of the prostate and the cancers that grow tend to invade these glands first. One of the principles of any cancer surgery is that all tissue within a half an inch of the cancer should be cut out to ensure all the cancer cells are removed. This lessens the chances of metastasis (spreading) or recurrence (return) of the cancer resulting from the growth of cancer cells that were left behind. As you can see, the rectum is also immediately adjacent to the prostate but cannot be removed. Fortunately, because of the developmental anatomy of the prostate, there is a special protective layer called Denonvillier's facia between the rectum

SURGERY FOR A CANCEROUS VERSUS A NON-CANCEROUS PROSTATE

Surgeries done for non-cancerous (benign) prostate diseases are called "simple" prostatectomies, as opposed to "radical" prostatectomies done to treat prostate cancer. In a simple prostatectomy for benign disease, only the inner enlarged tissue of the prostate is removed and the shell of the prostate and seminal vesicles are left intact, as shown in Figure 2.1. Simple prostatectomies are done to reduce or eliminate symptoms of BPH (*see* page 5) that cause a man to run to the bathroom frequently and urgently. Surgery can help correct these symptoms; in fact, for many years, surgery to treat benign enlargement of the prostate was the most common operation done by urologists.

However, the invention and success of various pills that can either shrink (Avodart and Proscar, generic- finasteride) or relax the prostate to increase the urinary flow (Flomax, Uroxatrol, Rapaflow, generic: prazosin) have made simple prostatectomy a relatively uncommon operation.

If the medications do not work, there are now several different types of simple prostate procedures that can be done for BPH. An "open" operation is one done through an incision in the lower abdomen or the perineum. Simple prostatectomies may also be "transurethral," done by introducing an instrument through the urethra to remove or alter the tissue around the urethra (this is called trans-urethral resection of the prostate [TURP]). It is important to remember that even if the removed tissue is benign, a cancer can develop in the shell of the gland in the small amount of prostate tissue left behind after a simple prostatectomy. Another common method of treating BPH is by burning the tissue with a laser beam. Unlike the TURP no tissue specimen is sent for examination to the pathologist. Therefore, if you have had a simple prostatectomy or another form of minimally invasive prostate surgery such as a TURP, or especially if you have had laser treatment or transurethral microwave surgery, you must still continue to get annual rectal exams of the prostate and PSA tests.

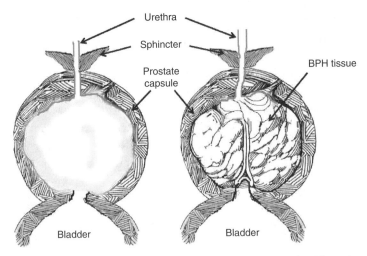

Figure 2.1 The prostate gland with enlarged, non-cancerous, tissue (BPH) on the right. During surgery for benign disease, only the enlarged tissue is removed and the capsule of the prostate is left behind, as shown on the left side of the diagram. The seminal vesicles are not seen during a benign operation and are left behind. The cavity left after removal of the benign tissue shrinks but the space left as the prostatic urethra is larger than would be present in the normal prostate without surgery. (Courtesy of Kelvin Davies, Ph.D.)

A PATIENT'S STORY: A SIMPLE PROSTATECTOMY TURNS NOT-SO-SIMPLE

At age 70, Simon B. was having great difficulty emptying his bladder and found that he needed to urinate every hour, day and night. On one occasion, he had a fever of 104 degrees with shaking chills and was diagnosed with a urinary tract infection that probably resulted from his not emptying his bladder of urine after each trip to the bathroom. Examination by his urologist showed that his prostate had grown to 130 g—more than five times his normal 25 g. His PSA was not elevated and cancer was not suspected. He had a simple open prostatectomy, and over a few months all of the abnormal urinary symptoms disappeared. All of the tissue reviewed was found to be benign with no suspicion of cancer. Simon was advised to return for annual visits but did not do so.

Five years later, his family doctor obtained a PSA and found a result of 28 ng/mL: more than five times normal. At that time, Simon returned to the urologist and rectal exam revealed a very hard prostate. A biopsy showed the presence of an aggressive, Gleason's 8 cancer. Scans showed no evidence of metastatic disease. Now 75 years old and in otherwise good health, Simon was advised to have EBRT and androgen deprivation therapy (ADT) for the best chance of cure or control of the cancer. A year later, Simon is still on hormone therapy and his PSA has stayed steady at 0.0 ng/mL, which indicates that the cancer is under control.

and prostate that prevents spread of prostate cancer into the rectum in all but the most advanced cases.

There are two basic "approaches" or ways into the body to reach the prostate: either through the lower abdomen or between the scrotum and the anus. Most commonly (96% of the time), the surgeon makes an incision through the lower abdomen, south of the belly button and north of the pubic bone; this is called a retropubic incision. Prostate surgery done this way is called a radical retropubic prostatectomy. In the second surgical approach, called a radical perineal prostatectomy, the incision is made between the anus and the scrotum (the sac that contains the testicles) in an area called the perineum. This is a more direct route yet is currently less common—only 4% of prostatectomies are done through the perineum—because most urological surgeons have not been trained in the approach.

Your Anatomy: Before and After Surgery

It is important to understand what happens during a radical prostatectomy to be prepared for the changes that will occur after the prostate is removed.

The prostate gland is important for men who want to have children. Once men are past the desire to father children, it is an organ that is not strictly necessary for normal daily living. Its function during reproductive years is to make fluid that help keep sperm alive after the ejaculation of the seminal fluid. Only about 1% of the seminal fluid volume is sperm, the rest is liquid generated by the prostate gland and the seminal vesicles. So after removal of the prostate, when a man has sex, he will still have orgasm and all the good feelings that happen with sex, but he will not have the emission of any fluid. That means that during post-prostatectomy sex, he will "shoot blanks" or have dry orgasms.

The prostate gland sits between the bladder and the urethra, the tube through which men pass urine and semen. The seminal vesicles (that make half of the seminal fluid) are attached to the back lower portion of the prostate. In a good cancer operation, they must be removed along with the prostate because the cancer cells can grow into those glands where they are attached. After the prostate and seminal vesicles are removed, there is a space of a few inches between the bladder opening and the urethra. The surgeon must reattach the urethra directly to the bladder. That joining, called anastomosis, is critical to rapid healing and control of urine. This joining is held in place with a few sutures while they heal together; usually these stitches dissolve in a few weeks. Figure 2.2 shows the anatomy of the prostate area before (2.2a), during (2.2b), and after (2.2c) surgery.

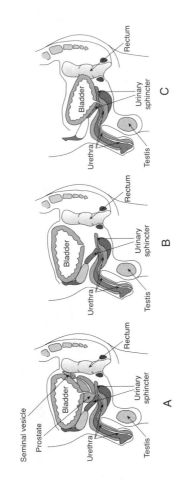

Figure 2.2 The change in anatomy associated with radical prostatectomy. Panel A shows the relationship of the organs before surgery. Panel B shows the relationship during the surgery after the prostate and seminal vesicles have been removed but before the bladder is reconnected. Panel C shows the anatomy after the bladder is joined to the sphincter, creating a continuous urinary tract. (Courtesy of Kelvin Davies, Ph.D.)

Thanks to technological advances in recent years, there are several different surgical techniques of radical prostatectomies to consider when choosing a cancer treatment.

Radical Retropubic Prostatectomy

In the 1980s, researchers discovered that the nerves that control penile erections lay adjacent to the prostate and could be swept aside easily when approached from this side during surgery, thus sparing the nerves and theoretically preserving erectile ability. This breakthrough gave men hope that they could have normal erections after their prostatectomy and still be potentially cured of their cancer. Radical prostatectomies became more acceptable treatments and, as the number of these surgeries performed grew, surgeons became more skilled and the surgical techniques became more and more advanced. Most urologists have experience with the radical retropubic prostatectomy. With this surgery, an incision is made in the abdomen from the belly button down to the pubic area, as shown in Figure 2.3.

There are several advantages of this approach. First, as a long-established procedure, most urologists are comfortable and confident in their ability to perform it. Second, the nerve-sparing approach increases the likelihood of sexual potency post-operatively. (This is true for any of the other surgeries, which usually have a better outcome for potency than radiation.)

However, there are also some disadvantages to the radical retropubic prostatectomy, including the potential for large blood loss resulting from the concentration of blood vessels in the region just around the prostate. In addition, there tends to be a longer recovery time than with some other approaches because of a larger incision and blood loss. Despite the nerve-sparing approach, patients still have a 50% chance of impotence and a 10% chance of urinary incontinence after recovery.[1]

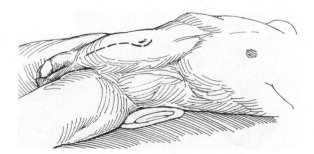

Figure 2.3 The position of the patient and the incision that is used for an open retropubic radical prostatectomy. (Courtesy of Kelvin Davies, Ph.D.)

Laparoscopic Radical Prostatectomy

The next prostatectomy approach developed was the laparoscopic radical prostatectomy. During that operation, the surgeon makes a small incision near the bellybutton, and inserts a small video camera attached to a flexible tube that contains a fiber-optic light and a magnifying lens into the patient's abdomen. Carbon dioxide gas is pushed into the abdomen, inflating it to create a dome-like working space with room for the camera and surgical instruments. Then, watching each move through the magnified video image, the surgeon inserts instruments through several small openings in the abdomen, and removes the prostate and seminal vesicles in a manner similar to the traditional radical retropubic operation. It is sort of like doing surgery using chopsticks from the outside of the body. The prostate and seminal vesicles are removed through a separate small incision in the lower abdomen.

The laparoscopic method takes longer then the regular radical retropubic operation but has less bleeding because the pressure of the CO_2 gas on the veins compresses them and keeps them from bleeding. There is also less post-operative pain because there are several small incisions rather than one large one.

NERVE-SPARING SURGERY

One of the greatest innovations in prostate surgery has been the ability to spare the nerves that run on either side of the prostate. These nerves are important to urinary and sexual function, and damaging them can lead to erectile dysfunction (ED) or bladder problems. When nerves on both sides of the prostate are saved, it is called a bilateral nerve-sparing prostatectomy. When only one side can be spared, it is called a unilateral nerve-sparing prostatectomy. Unfortunately, not all prostatectomies are nerve-sparing (see Table 2.2).

As you can see in Figure 2.4, there are a tremendous number of nerves in this area and sometimes, the location or extent of the cancer makes it impossible to spare all the nerves. It can be more difficult to spare the nerves in obese men, men who have had prior pelvic infections or surgery, or men who have already had radiation. Because nerves are very difficult to see (they look like light fishing lines), a procedure such as a robotic assisted prostatectomy (*see* below) can be a good choice, as it offers a magnified view of the area. Some surgeons believe in removing all the nerves if the tumor appears to be near the capsule of the prostate. The issue of nerve sparing is definitely one you should discuss with your surgeon before surgery.

Table 2.2. Nerve-Sparing Surgeries

Technique	Percent of surgeries that are nerve-sparing[a,b]
Radical retropubic	71% to 90%
Laparoscopic	38% to 100%
Robotic-assisted	60% to 97%

[a] Berryhill R, Jr., Jhaveri J, Yadav R, Leung R, Rao S, El-Hakim A, et al. Robotic prostatectomy: a review of outcomes compared with laparoscopic and open approaches. *Urology* 2008; 72(1):15–23.

[b] Krumholtz JS, Carvalhal GF, Ramos CG, Smith DS, Thorson P, Yan Y, et al. Prostate-specific antigen cutoff of 2.6 ng/mL for prostate cancer screening is associated with favorable pathologic tumor features. *Urology* 2002; 60(3):469–473.

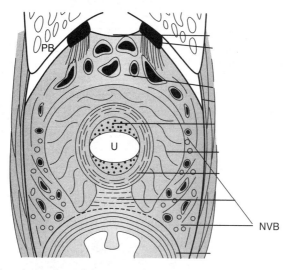

Figure 2.4 The relationship of the nerves (neurovascular bundle [NVB]) that control erection to the apical end (the end near the urethra) of the prostate. The prostate is the grey-shaded area; the urethra is the white oval marked "U" in the center; the black shapes are nerve bundles.

(Reprinted with permission *European Urology*. Copyright © 2010, Elsevier.)

Robotic-Assisted Radical Prostatectomy

The robotic-assisted radical prostatectomy has virtually supplanted the laparoscopic prostatectomy. Only a few years old, this new technology combines the laparoscopic approach—using an intra-abdominal video camera and CO_2 gas—with a multi-armed robot (called DaVinci) that can manipulate many surgical instruments at once. It is almost like a prostatectomy video game, but it's a real patient and a real surgery. The surgeon conducts the operation by

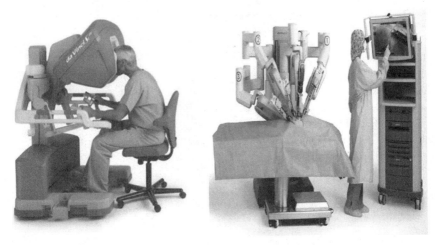

Figure 2.5 The surgeon is sitting at the 3D television consol on the left. He uses the lever and pedals to control the arms of the robot. The diagram on the right shows the robot positioned over the patient. One or two assistants are needed to change the instruments and care for the lens with the camera seated on one of the arms.
The assistants watch the surgery on the HD television monitor.
(Reprinted with permission by Intuitive Surgical, Inc. © 2010 Intuitive Surgical, Inc.)

watching a 3D monitor that streams live video from the camera inside the patient (*see* Figure 2.5). The surgeon's hands manipulate the robot controls at a desk across the room while the robotic hands in the abdomen perform the operation at the surgeon's instructions. Nurses and other attendants also follow the surgery's progress from video monitors. In the future, the technology could allow a doctor to operate on a person in a different hospital or in another city.

The advantage of the robotic prostatectomy is that the surgeon has a clear, magnified view of the patient's interior, which minimizes the chances of surgical error. Another advantage is the rotation ability of the robot arms allows for very precise suturing so that the joining of the bladder to the urethra is more accurate and there is less chance of urine leaking out with subsequent scarring.

> *"My father died of prostate cancer, so when I was diagnosed, I wanted it out and I wanted it out now. The idea of waiting to see what might happen was so distasteful. I just wanted to get it done with and let the healing begin."*
>
> —Jake T.

The disadvantages are mainly that it may be difficult to find. The surgeon must go through special training to use the robot in addition to their surgical and medical school training. Also, the cost of the machine to the hospital may mean this approach is not available to all patients, depending on their location and health insurance coverage.

The Radical Perineal Prostatectomy

The radical perineal prostatectomy is the oldest of the surgical methods for removing the prostate. In this approach, with the man lying on his back with his legs pulled back, the incision is made between the scrotum and the anus, which is in close proximity to the prostate (*see* Figure 2.6).

It often can be done successfully in men who are not candidates for surgery with other anatomic approaches, such as obese men who have a very large belly, people who have already had extensive lower abdominal surgery, and men who have had a kidney transplant. In each of those examples, it is nearly impossible to approach the prostate through the lower abdomen.

I often recommend perineal surgery for all my patients because it can be done rapidly (within 70 to 90 minutes) and with little bleeding. In general, you want your surgery to be over quickly, because the longer you are under general anesthesia, the higher the chance of complications. Also, a quicker surgery can mean a shorter recovery time. From a surgeon's point of view, the perineal approach also provides a better angle to view the bladder and urethral area after the removal of the prostate gland. As mentioned earlier, the surgeon must carefully reattach the urethra directly to the bladder; the successful joining (called *anastomosis*) is critical to rapid healing and control of urine. Because that

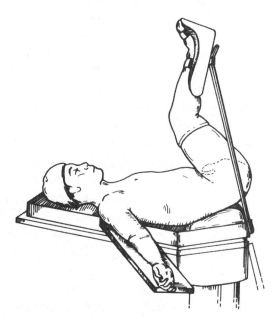

Figure 2.6 The exaggerated lithotomy position that allows the radical perineal surgery to be done.
(Reprinted with permission from *J Urology*. Copyright © 2004, Elsevier.)

anatomy is in direct view in the perineal approach, the anastomosis is relatively easy to do. The possibility of urine leakage and the complication of bladder neck contracture (*see* page 93) are less likely.

The disadvantage of the operation is that it requires a surgeon highly experienced in perineal anatomy and training to do the removal. Most training centers in the United States do not train their young surgeons to do that approach, and there are only a limited number of surgeons available throughout the country. Therefore, only about 4% of radical prostatectomies in the United States are done with that anatomical approach.

Choosing a Surgical Treatment

When you and your doctor have decided that surgery is the best choice to treat your prostate cancer, the next question is which method to choose. The outcome from each approach can be equally satisfactory, so much depends on the individual circumstances. If the man has pre-existing conditions, they may dictate a certain choice. For example, as mentioned above, men with prior abdominal surgeries, morbid obesity (300 pounds or more), or a kidney transplant would be wise to choose a perineal prostatectomy.

In general, the robotic and perineal procedures have a shorter time in the hospital and a shorter recovery time, as those surgeries require smaller incisions and usually less time under anesthesia than the radical retropubic. Whether or not you retain potency is more often a matter of the surgeon's expertise and the location and size of the cancer than a particular surgical approach. Your unique anatomy also plays a role as the nerves can be in slightly different positions in different people, and on some people more than others, it may be harder for the surgeon to avoid touching them or possibly nicking them when removing the cancerous tissue. Because nerves don't show up on scans, this is one of the factors that the surgeon faces in the operating room, and thus cannot predict with absolute certainty whether there will be any nerve damage in your case. (For more information on what can cause ED after surgery, *see* page 51.) For those particularly concerned about urinary continence after surgery, I might steer them toward robotic or perineal surgeries as these afford the best possible view of the urethral-bladder area so the surgeon can have the best possible chance of joining the urethra and bladder tightly and smoothly. However, I would say that the surgeon him- or herself is a more important factor in a successful outcome than which procedure is used.

If there aren't specific medical or insurance reasons to choose a particular approach, then my suggestion is to consider the experience of the surgeon and the surgical team as well as the hospital. Robotic surgery may not be available in your area, and then you would have to decide if you are willing to travel to have that procedure. Depending on your support network and transportation options, that may or may not be possible. Remember there will be follow-up appointments with the same doctor. A good doctor is worth traveling for, if you are able. Make certain that you and your surgeon relate well to each other—should you have a complication you want a medical team that you feel good about. Then make certain that you know his qualifications. A surgeon doing his third robotic prostatectomy or doing only one surgery a month is unlikely to get the same results as an experienced operator who does one or two radical prostatectomies (or more) a week by whatever method.

QUESTIONS FOR THE SURGEON

In the stressful time after your diagnosis, it can be hard to ask questions during your appointments—especially when the doctor is busy relaying a lot of information to you. However, there are several important questions to ask your surgeon before agreeing to a procedure:

1. What is their experience with different prostatectomies? How many do they do a week or month? How many years of experience do they have with this procedure?
2. Why did they choose their particular method over other approaches?
3. Is he or she board-certified in urology? What special training do they have, such as a fellowship or extensive experience in their residency or practice?
4. What are the chances that the nerves can be spared in your situation?
5. Make certain, by asking the surgeon, that a radical prostatectomy is a common operation in the hospital to which you will be admitted. If only a few per month or year are done there, then that is not good for you. You want to be operated on in a hospital with the latest equipment and operating room personnel that know how to use them.

It is a good idea to see more than one surgeon, so you can compare their answers.

Try not to be swayed by the marketing hype of some hospitals and physicians. If the doctor tells you that none of his patients have complications and he has a 100% success rate, go to someone else because he must sell used cars on the side. Do not be afraid to seek other opinions or to travel to get what you want. Although I believe in most circumstances that your surgeon and hospital should be conveniently close for family and follow-up care, you have only one life and you should be diligent about taking care of it.

Recovery from Surgery

Recovery from a radical prostatectomy is usually straightforward for most men, depending on their overall health. In the weeks or months leading up to the operation, I usually suggest increasing the amount of exercise, such as walking or swimming, to be as strong as possible going into surgery. The physical training will help with breathing and muscle tone and perhaps will help you to lose a few unnecessary pounds of weight—all of which will help your recovery. There are other exercises that may prove even more important to your recovery: pelvic floor exercises. When started in the weeks before surgery, these exercises can help your body regain urinary continence faster after the prostate is removed (*see* page 99).

In today's insurance-dominated medical world, men will be discharged from the hospital either the same day, or no more than 3 days after surgery. Medically, there is little that must be done at home during the recuperation time. For any adult person undergoing a surgical procedure, it takes at least 6 weeks to return to a normal, pre-operative energy level. Men who have the laparoscopic, robotic, or perineal surgery can return to work and daily living faster—usually within 2 weeks—because there is less pain with the smaller incisions. With a traditional radical retropubic procedure, it might take the full 6 weeks.

While the bladder-to-urethra joining is healing, a catheter must be in place to drain urine from the bladder. A catheter is a flexible tube inserted into the urethra to drain the urine so that the muscles in that area do not move, which could disturb the stitches. The catheter is threaded into the penis before surgery, and most surgeons leave the catheter in place for about a week after surgery. The catheter is often uncomfortable to wear but a necessary component of the operation. A small fluid-filled balloon on the bladder side of the catheter keeps the catheter in place until the surgeon removes the catheter, a procedure that can be painlessly and easily completed in the doctor's office. During the day, the catheter can be attached to a draining leg bag so that the men can leave the house and move about normally. This bag will need to be emptied by you into the toilet when it becomes full, but otherwise the catheter requires little care by the patient—just gentle cleaning of the area to lower the risk of infection.

After the catheter is removed, most men will go through a period of time when they leak urine. The bulk of the prostate helps with urinary control, and when it is suddenly removed, other muscles must assume a greater role in urinary continence. The two muscles that affect the control of urine are the bladder neck, which is not under your voluntary control, and the external urinary sphincter. The latter muscle can shut off the urinary flow while you are urinating. To help with control of the starting and stopping of urination, the muscle needs to be strengthened as if you were weight-lifting. The more lifting, the stronger the muscle. Of course there are no tiny weights to lift, but muscle strength can be increased with repetitive exercise like a Kegel exercise. The best program is starting and stopping the urinary stream. This can be started long before surgery. Each time you urinate, stop the stream several times. That action will increase the strength and size of the sphincter muscle and help with control after the surgery. (*See* Chapters 5 and 6 for a detailed discussion of urinary incontinence and what to do about it.)

Possible Post-Operative Problems

The changes that can occur after surgery—although common for most prostate cancer patients, no matter what their treatments—can be trying. Each post-operative patient faces some challenges, whether large or small, because of the removal of the prostate gland. Some have suggested doing a less aggressive "lumpectomy" surgery for prostate cancer, as is done for women with breast cancer, so that only a portion of the gland is removed as a means of reducing post-treatment complications. However unlike breast cancer, prostate cancer is multifocal—that is, it may be present in many areas of the gland at the same time. Because some tumors (groups of cancer cells) can be so tiny that they are not detectable, the surgeon may not know what areas to remove and which to leave behind. Moreover, the prostate is located deep in the pelvis, unlike the breast, and is difficult to approach with repeated surgeries, should it be necessary to re-operate to remove additional cancer cells. Also, the diagnostic imaging tests (X-ray, magnetic resonance imaging [MRI], computed tomography [CT]) needed to locate tumors are not sensitive enough to detect very small or microscopic tumors.

The two most common complications that can occur after surgery for radical prostatectomy are erectile dysfunction and urinary incontinence. Following a nerve-sparing radical prostatectomy, a man can have normal sex drive (libido) and may be able to achieve no, partial, or full erection. And most men (about 80%) are able to have orgasms (the pleasurable sensation that happens with sexual activity), although there will not be ejaculation of semen, because the organs responsible for ejaculatory fluids have been removed. Erectile dysfunction will occur in most men for a brief time after surgery, but if it is a lasting problem, it could be because nerves were nicked or moved during surgery and may take longer to heal, or they may not heal at all. There is still hope for regaining potency in both situations—Chapters 3 and 4 will address post-operative ED and its treatment in detail.

Incontinence can be a devastating complication of radical cancer treatment. After surgery, most men have some incontinence after the catheter is removed;

unfortunately, urinary incontinence persists in up to 15% of men 2 years after surgery. The incidence of the incontinence is higher among older men who have surgery. Researchers are not sure why older men are more affected; it could be because older men have lost some muscle mass or nerve endings or that they are more likely to have pre-existing bladder problems that are only "revealed" once the prostate is removed (*see* page 88). After prostatectomy is done and the prostate gland is removed, the anatomy of a man's urinary system changes. The prostate sits between the bladder and urethra and helps control the flow of urine, preventing leakage out of the bladder when the pressure in the bladder is high. When the prostate gland is completely removed, as happens with radical prostatectomy, that buffer is also removed and control of urine leakage becomes dependent on the muscles of the pelvic floor, known as the

---

A PATIENT'S STORY: A TYPICAL PROSTATECTOMY

Wayne T. was a 60-year-old man whose PSA went from 4.1 to 5.4 in 1 year. I performed a biopsy that confirmed that Wayne had localized prostate cancer, with a Gleason's score of 7. His health was good, and he chose to have a radical perineal prostatectomy.

As is typical with this surgery, he was admitted to the hospital the morning of the operation. The surgery went well and after about 2 hours, he was back in the recovery room, where he had some pain medication. Luckily he did not require any pain medications thereafter. We left a small drain in his perineum (to remove any blood or urine), which we removed the following morning. The Foley catheter was draining pinkish urine from his urethra, which is normal post-operatively. He was discharged to go home about 48 hours after he arrived at the hospital.

One week later, he returned to my office to have the catheter removed. As is typical after radical prostatectomy, when the catheter was out, he occasionally leaked some urine without being able to control it. He was instructed to do the pelvic floor (Kegel) exercises as much as possible. Another concern he had was moving his bowels, as he was afraid of possible pain and damaging the surgical sutures. I advised him to use stool softeners (such as colace) and to eat fiber-rich food and drink plenty of water.

At his 6-week post-operative visit, Wayne was still leaking urine. I reassured him and encouraged him to persist with the exercises. After 3 months he had total urinary control—this is about the typical length of time it takes most men to regain continence. He proudly told me that he had resumed work 2 weeks after surgery and began playing golf again after a month.

---

external urinary sphincter. By strengthening this muscle, you can lower your chances of post-operative incontinence, or if you strengthen post-surgery, you will increase your chances of returning to full continence.

NON-SURGICAL TREATMENTS FOR PROSTATE CANCER

Of the non-surgical treatments for localized prostate cancer, the most common is radiation treatment, which burns out the cancer with targeted doses of radiation. About 40% of the men who are diagnosed with prostate cancer undergo either radiation or have radiation combined with surgery. Watchful waiting is another treatment option also employed (temporarily) by certain populations of patients (about 10% of the total men with prostate cancer). Hormone therapy is another treatment, mainly used in cases of non-localized cancer (*see* Chapter 8 for more information on hormone therapy).

Keeping an Eye on it: Watchful Waiting and Active Surveillance

There are two treatments that involve not immediately treating the prostate cancer but, rather, watching it: watchful waiting and active surveillance. These options are not for every patient but can be the best choice for certain people.

WATCHFUL WAITING
Watchful waiting is the deliberate act of identifying the presence of a cancer with a biopsy and then making a bet. The bet is that the tumor will grow slowly enough so that some other disease, or even just plain old age, will be the eventual cause of death of that person—and not the newly identified cancer. This can be the best choice of action if the patient is very elderly or already experiencing serious health problems. The medical consensus is that if you expect to live less than 10 years, you may consider not treating the prostate cancer and instead just keep an eye on it. In general, watchful waiting should only be used for men with localized cancer (if it has spread already, it should be treated so as to buy the patient as much time as possible). For a generally healthy, younger man, however, this can be a very risky route to choose.

ACTIVE SURVEILLANCE
Active surveillance is slightly different; the surgeon and the patient agree that they will monitor the disease with the expectation that curative therapy will begin if the cancer appears to progress. To be a candidate for active surveillance,

the patient must meet certain criteria (as in a study from the Royal Marsden Hospital in London):[2]

- Ages between 50 and 80 years
- Gleason's score less than or equal to 7
- Clinical stage T1 or T2 disease
- Total PSA less than 15
- PSA score doubling time less than 2 years
- 50% or less of the biopsy samples positive for cancer
- A reasonable state of health with no other major medical problems

As is true for most cancers, prostate cancer in its early stages usually causes few problems and grows silently and slowly. However, once the cancer begins to reach a certain size, urinary symptoms such as urgency, frequency, bleeding, and infection can occur as the growing tumor blocks the outflow of urine from the bladder. Patients being treated with surveillance should be sure they keep their doctors informed of these or similar symptoms so they can decide whether or not non-intervention is still the best choice.

Advocates of active surveillance believe that so-called "clinically insignificant" (i.e., localized, less aggressive) prostate cancer is overtreated and over-diagnosed and that treatment of these cancers can have a significant adverse effect to the patient's quality of life. For active surveillance to be successful, the patient must agree to careful follow-up, including repeat biopsies and blood tests every year. About 50% of the men go on to have actual treatment, some because of rapid increase of PSA, an upgrading of the Gleason's score, or patient preference.

Those opposed to active surveillance emphasize that there is currently no way to discover which cancers will grow and which will not: One in every four men who undergo active surveillance should not have done so because their cancer progresses while they wait. They also believe that there is no uniformly accurate way to follow the progression of disease—that is, some patients may see another rise in PSA over a period of a year or two; others may rise suddenly over a month or two. There is also no way of knowing if the cancer will still be curable if it progresses. Opponents to active surveillance cite a study showing that 25% of men who chose active surveillance developed metastatic cancer (their cancer spread outside the prostate) within a few years.[3,4,5,6] There are no published long-term studies that prove whether men under active surveillance who go on to active therapy are harmed by the delay. However, patients should consider that if they wait to treat the cancer until the tumor grows, the bigger tumor may mean either an increased risk of side effects (because it requires more extensive surgery) or it may mean a shift from curable to incurable disease.

Because all prostate cancers will grow, the choice of surveillance depends on both known and unknown factors. The age of the patient and the aggressiveness (grade) and extent (stage) of the tumor are the most important factors. Certainly a 75-year-old man with diabetes and high blood pressure with a low-grade, small, non-aggressive tumor is more likely to die as a result of a heart attack or stroke than from prostate cancer. The opposite is true for an otherwise healthy 50-year-old, who is likely to be around for many years—plenty of time for the prostate cancer to grow and spread.

Radiation Treatment

Radiation therapy can be used to cure localized prostate cancer or, if it is used in conjunction with surgery or hormone therapy, to cure or control a non-localized cancer. Radiation energy damages the cancer cells' DNA so that they do not reproduce and causes the cells to die more rapidly. Radiation energy affects all of the cells into which the radiation beam enters, and if the cancer cells are more sensitive (i.e., they die more easily than a normal cell), the treatment can be very effective. If the cancer cell is equally or less affected by the radiation than a normal cell, then the radiation needs to be very carefully guided to the cancer to ensure effective treatment. Because prostate cancer cells can be relatively resistant to radiation, high doses of energy are often used to kill the prostate cancer. Unfortunately these dosages can also cause damage to normal cells in the rectum and bladder. Techniques have continued to improve over the years, and many researchers in this field are still working to improve the delivery of radiation to the prostate gland itself without damaging nearby tissue. Unlike surgery, the overall anatomy and relationship to the nearby organs is unchanged after radiation, but in the long term, the prostate may become smaller and more rigid as radiation can cause scar tissue to develop.

Types of Radiation

There are three methods of administering radiation for prostate cancer: external beam radiation (EBRT), brachytherapy (radiation seeds left in temporarily or permanently), and a combination therapy. You and your doctor will discuss which approach would be most effective for you, depending on the size of your prostate and the size of the cancer (as estimated by the biopsy and imaging studies like CT scan or MRI), the aggressiveness of the cancer, the location of your cancer in the prostate, your doctor's area of expertise, and other diagnostic studies. In general, those with bigger tumors are probably more likely to be cured with EBRT (or combination therapy) because the radiation is not confined in one small place like a seed but, rather, covers a little more area. (A little bit of imprecision is not a bad thing if you don't know exactly where the outlying cancer cells are.) The more benign tumors may have a better chance of cure with the seeds.

External Beam Radiation

In the EBRT method, the patient lies on a table and the radiation beam is delivered for several minutes to a specific area as mapped out by computer. This computer mapping for precise delivery of the radiation is accomplished during a "treatment simulation session" done by CT scanning prior to treatment. An MRI might also be requested to help plan the attack. Together, these scans tell the doctor the exact coordinates of the tumor and affected areas so that the radiation is aimed directly at the target.

The treatment is usually given 5 days a week, for 6 to 10 weeks, until a predetermined dose of radiation is given. Before the EBRT is started, many men are given an injection to limit the production of the male hormone testosterone for up to 2 years before, during, and after treatment. The therapy, known as androgen deprivation therapy (ADT), is done to shrink the tumor and the prostate to make the radiation more effective. Some centers give the ADT only for specific grades of cancer. (*See* Chapter 8 for more discussion of ADT.)

Some radiation therapy centers use a special CT scan and computer to deliver more precisely aimed radiation beams. This capability is known as three-dimensional conformal radiation therapy (3D-CRT). The use of 3D-CRT appears to reduce the chance of injury to nearby body structures, including the bladder and rectum. Because 3D-CRT can better target the area of cancer, radiation oncologists are evaluating whether higher doses of radiation can be given safely to achieve greater cure rates. Preliminary data from several cancer programs suggest that the higher radiation dose delivered with 3D-CRT can reduce the rate of local cancer recurrence.

The latest mode of EBRT is called intensity-modulated radiation therapy (IMRT), which uses a computer-controlled process for delivering the radiation beam. The method maximizes the amount of radiation given to the cancer while minimizing surrounding tissue destruction or injury. In IMRT treatment, the radiation beams enter the body from multiple angles and higher doses, converging on the prostate. Thus the highest levels of radiation are delivered to the prostate, and the areas of radiation exposure outside of the prostate are lower. However, the surrounding levels are not zero, as some nerves and blood vessels that go to the penis are still in the field of radiation. Two new markers to better improve the radiation therapy may be used in some centers. Each requires a separate instillation of a small device near the prostate. The first called Calypso emits an electromagnetic beam that precisely localizes the prostate even when you breathe during the radiation treatment. The second called dose verification system (DVS) monitors exactly how much radiation has been given to the prostate. These devices were approved by FDA in 2006 so long term results that compare their use to older treatments are not yet available. Similarly, the Cyberknife system of delivering radiation uses the prior placement of five gold seeds around the prostate to mark its location during the therapy. Proton beam therapy is another form of extremely precise radiation historically used for treating brain and head and neck tumors, where precision is extremely important. It is not clear that that degree of precision is an advantage in treating prostate cancers, particularly because the prostate moves during the treatment.

External beam treatment is usually painless—most patients complain more of the tedium of daily visits than of pain. Other than the interruption to your daily routine, there are few immediate repercussions of treatment, as it takes a while for any side effects to appear after radiation. Urinary incontinence is less likely than with surgery, as a general rule, but ED can be worse (depending on which study's numbers you use; *see* Table 2.3 on page 45). Unlike surgery, there is a risk of inflammation from the radiation in the surrounding organs (the bladder and rectum), which can cause urinary urgency and frequency and rectal pain and bleeding for several weeks after the treatment. These side effects are discussed in Chapter 7.

Prostate Seeds or Brachytherapy

In brachytherapy, the patient receives his radiation dose through metallic "seeds" that are placed in the prostate to kill the cancer. There are two methods of brachytherapy available.

The first and most commonly administered form is a one-time treatment done under anesthesia as an outpatient in the hospital. Working together, a urologist and a radiotherapist plant 50 to 100 "seeds" in the patient's prostate. The radiotherapist designs a treatment map that shows where the urologist must place the radiation dose to reach the cancer cells without extending into any nearby tissue. The patient lies in the lithotomy position: on his back with

---

Lithotomy is derived from the Greek *lithos,* or stone, and *otomy,* to cut out. It is the position developed by surgeons in the 1700s to cure a common problem, in that time, of bladder stones, before the development of anesthesia. The surgeons had to be very fast and were able to remove the stones in less than a minute.

---

his legs raised up in stirrups. For brachytherapy, the legs are not pulled back as far as is done for a radical perineial prostatectomy. An ultrasound probe is placed in the rectum and the image is used to guide the placement of hollow needles into the prostate. The seeds are sent into the prostate via these hollow needles.

The metallic seeds to which the radioactivity has been added, each about the size of a rice grain, are placed into the prostate tissue and left in the prostate permanently to give a continual dose of radiation. Two types of seeds can be used by the radiotherapist. One, Iodine 125, gives a low dose over 300 days. The other, palladium, gives a higher dose over 85 days. The patient can return home in a day or two. Some patients have difficulty urinating after this form of therapy and may require the placement of a catheter or additional medication to help them urinate.

To receive this treatment, the patient must have a prostate gland that is no larger than about 50 g, or twice the normal size of the prostate. This size limitation exists to ensure that all regions of the prostate will receive sufficient radiation to kill the cancer.

The other form of brachytherapy is called high-dose rate (HDR) brachytherapy and is used much less commonly and only to treat aggressive forms of cancer. In this treatment, 18 to 25 small plastic tubes are placed in the prostate and the radiation seeds are placed into the tubes. A computer-controlled machine then pushes another type of radioactive seed called Iridium into the prostate, which is left in place for a short time (several hours). The computer controls how long the seeds are left in place and then the entire plastic tube is removed, along with the seeds. During the treatment the man is on bedrest in the hospital overnight. This type of therapy is usually given along with EBRT and possibly with hormone therapy.

Combination Therapy
The third form of radiation is a combination of seeds and EBRT. This type of therapy is done for men who have "high-risk" disease (*see* Table 2.1 on page 20). In this case, the seeds are placed first and the EBRT given afterward. The reason for the combination is to treat tumors that are believed to have already extended outside of the prostate into the local tissues. This combination treatment may also be suggested for tumors that are thought to be more aggressive and therefore more resistant to standard radiation treatment.

Another form of combination therapy is called adjuvant—it is additional therapy given to lower the risk that the cancer will come back. The most commonly used adjuvant therapies are radiation and hormone therapy. Adjuvant therapy is usually given in a man who, after surgery, was found to have a cancer extending out of the prostate into the seminal vesicles or bladder neck.

A PATIENT'S STORY: A TYPICAL RADIATION TREATMENT

Glenn W. is a 72-year-old man with an elevated PSA of 6 and a Gleason's score of 6. Several years earlier, he had suffered a mild heart attack but was now well enough to receive general anesthesia. His prostate was measured at 45 g (nearly double the normal size). However, he was urinating satisfactorily, waking only twice per night while taking an alpha-blocker (such as Flomax). He and his wife were not sexually active. He underwent placement of Iridium seeds as an outpatient procedure and was sent home the same day with a catheter in place. The catheter was removed 48 hours later in the doctor's office and he urinated without difficulty. For about 6 weeks after the seed placement he suffered from increased urination (every 2 hours) and had to wake up four or more times a night to urinate. The symptoms lasted for about 6 weeks and then he returned to his pre-seed state. His PSA dropped to a level of 2 and remained constant over the next year.

RECOVERY FROM RADIATION TREATMENT

Recovery from radiation is usually uneventful, especially for the first few months. There may some feelings of fatigue and rectal and bladder issues toward the end of the treatment. Because brachytherapy is done under anesthesia, there may be some issues from the anesthesia rather than any local irritation of the seeds. Routinely, anesthesia will cause people fatigue for up to 6 weeks until the adrenal hormones re-regulate themselves. So I recommend to my patients a gradual increase from no work, to part-time, then back to full-time work over a 6-week interval. Men can continue to work while receiving EBRT. Any irritative symptoms, such as difficulty urinating, may take several weeks after beginning EBRT to appear, and they will eventually diminish over several months.

Because you will have to return to your doctor at regular intervals to confirm that the treatment was effective, your doctor will be able to help ascertain which side effects are temporary nuisances and which (if any) are more serious cause for worry.

Possible Post-Radiation Problems

Because of the rectum and the bladder's proximity to the prostate, they almost always receive some of the radiation dose during the prostate treatment. As a result, the side effects from the two types of radiation primarily appear in those two organs. The immediate complications are irritation to the bladder and prostate that can cause increased urinary urgency and frequency and sometimes even urinary bleeding (gross, we know, but these things can happen). Those symptoms usually disappear within a few months. Of greater concern are changes to the rectum that cause pain, bleeding, and even fecal incontinence (involuntary loss of stool). Again, for most patients these symptoms are temporary.

A small number of men develop other radiation complications, such as scarring of the prostate that can cause it to narrow (called a stricture) and squeeze the urethra, making it difficult to urinate. Post-radiation stricture is a difficult problem to correct and usually requires surgery to open the channel. Because the radiation causes loss of blood supply to the prostate, the strictures can recur.

Over the long-term, men who have had radiation therapy may experience an increased occurrence of bladder and rectal cancers. Therefore, careful long-term follow-up is needed in any man who has been treated with radiation for prostate cancer. Of course, any man who has had treatment for prostate cancer should be followed in case the cancer recurs or continues to grow despite the full course of radiation.

After brachytherapy, the primary side effect is called acute radiation proctitis (proctitis is an inflammation of the lining of the rectum). Patients may experience the feeling of needing to go to the bathroom to have a bowel moment but nothing comes out, or they may have frequent or loose bowel movements, or bleeding from the rectum. They may also feel they have to urinate often, or with a sense of urgency. The most common of the symptoms is diarrhea, which occurs in 50% to 75% of the men who have brachytherapy. These complications usually last only a few months and then stop with no additional problems.

A number of men may develop chronic radiation proctitis 6 months to 2 years after the brachytherapy. It may occur in men who did not have acute radiation proctitis and is a more serious problem. It can cause rectal urgency, fecal incontinence, pain, rectal strictures, mucous discharge, and rectal bleeding. These problems stem from radiation damage to the small blood vessels of the rectal wall. The reported incidence of rectal complications ranges from 12% to 16% for mild problems (minimal, infrequent bleeding or clear mucous discharge not requiring medication), to 4% to 18% for intermediary problems (intermittent rectal bleeding not requiring pad use, diarrhea requiring medication) to 1% to 8% for significant problems (rectal bleeding requiring regular use of pads).

CHOOSING RADIATION AS A THERAPY

Knowing all that can go wrong, it can be difficult to make this (or any other treatment) choice. However, there are good reasons to pick radiation to treat prostate cancer. In my view, EBRT or seed therapy are better choices for those men who are not good surgery candidates or who do not wish to go through the stress of an operation. Older men, those with shorter life expectancies, and those with other medical problems are generally those who are smart to choose radiation therapy. For men who experience a recurrence of their cancer after surgery (meaning that some cancer cells remained in the body after surgery and reproduced), then radiation known as *salvage radiation* is the best course. There may be other cases, such as the example on page 19, when a patient's individual circumstances demand this choice.

COMPARING THERAPY CHOICES: SURVEYING THE NUMBERS

Faced with the need to decide between choices as varied as no therapy to an aggressive surgical intervention, some men rely on the advice of their physician, some shop around for advice from many physicians, some rely on the advice of family and friends, and some use the Internet for information. In addition to information concerning cure of the cancer, men and their partners also worry about the effect of the treatment upon quality of life, especially erectile function and urinary control.

The most useful advice in this situation would be accurate, clearly written scientific data that would state, "Using this specific treatment will give this result in x % of people." Unfortunately, no such specific help is available for several reasons. One reason is that there is no established uniform method to present outcome data that accurately compares results from one medical study, or even one hospital or one doctor, to another. What may be regarded as satisfactory erectile function to some researchers (or some patients) is abnormal to others. The rigidity of the penis, the duration of the erection, presence of a willing partner, sexual history, and desire for sex all contribute to the "normalcy" of the man, and few authors include all the details. Similarly, what defines urinary continence in some reports is the same as *incontinence* in others! The time men are evaluated after treatment is also variable—researchers describe much different outcomes if the results are compiled 6 months after treatment, rather than at 18 months.

Also, different medical centers take care of different patient populations. Because younger, healthier men with active sex lives have the best chance of more satisfactory outcomes for quality-of-life issues, wealthy medical centers with big budgets tend to court these types of patients through aggressive marketing. Obviously, doctors and hospitals that care for younger, healthier, wealthier, Caucasian men may report better outcomes than centers that care

A Patient's Story: Another Radiation Experience

Michael M. is a 70-year-old prostate cancer patient who underwent 2 months of EBRT for Stage 2 tumor. He had had no symptoms before his diagnosis, but during a routine physical, he discovered his PSA had doubled in a year. He chose to get a biopsy immediately instead of waiting another 6 months, and it turned out to be prostate cancer. "It was a shock. I thought of myself as a healthy person but it turned out I wasn't that healthy."

Michael originally planned to have surgery, but during his pre-operative check-up, his heart started "acting funny." So, he decided to not to put his heart through the stress of surgery and chose the radiation route instead. He went for EBRT therapy 5 days a week for just 10 minutes a visit. "I didn't mind the environment at all," Michael said, noting that the staff of his local medical center treated him with compassion and respect.

At first, he had no side effects, but gradually the radiation built up in his system and he did experience fatigue, frequent urination at night, diarrhea, and hemorrhoid flare-ups. Most of these problems went away in the month after he finished treatment. He credits his active lifestyle and his strong relationship network, including his wife of 40 years, for his resiliency. "During treatment, it was tough. I just tried to keep up with my routine as much as possible—swimming, taking art classes, seeing friends."

Michael's attitude probably helped him through, too. "It's been an eye-opening experience in a lot of ways." He admits to having anxiety about his upcoming blood tests that will determine how effective the EBRT was. But overall he says, "Thinking of myself as a cancer victim has passed. I'm grateful that there are treatments. There are people that have been cured, so that's hopeful."

for the poor, non-white populations who tend to have worse pre-cancer health care and less generous health insurance, and tend to be older, more obese, and have other illnesses—such as diabetes and hypertension—all of which can adversely affect their results.

So how can you find useful data? The best method to obtain helpful statistical information is to scan the literature—most of which is written in technical jargon with the numbers presented in a deliberately misleading way so as to make the results seem better, or more newsworthy, than they actually are. Table 2.3 is a summary of many reports, with the full range of results presented. The surgical results are for bilateral nerve-sparing surgery (meaning the nerves going down both sides of the prostate are spared). Results for unilateral nerve-sparing surgery (where the nerves on only one side are unscathed)

Table 2.3. TREATMENT TYPES AND OUTCOMES

	SURGERY			RADIATION	
	Radical retropubic	Laparoscopic	Robotic	External beam	Permanent seeds (I-125, Pd-103)
Erectile function preserved	22%–92%	43%–88%	33%–97%	28%–93%	49%–98%
Urinary continence preserved	60.5%–93%	60%–98%	82%–98%	92%	92%

are about 20% less than bilateral surgery for erectile function. In general, younger men (younger than 60 years old at time of treatment) can expect better results than men older than 65.

The data for urinary continence is obtained from several medical research papers that compared urinary function before and after cancer treatment. Another aspect in bladder and urinary concerns is what urination problems exist before the therapy. For example, a man with a large prostate with urinary high frequency and urgency pre-treatment may have a better outcome with surgery than after radiation therapy, because the troublesome prostate is removed. Radiation can cause more irritative symptoms like urgency and frequency, whereas surgery tends to cause problems with stress urinary incontinence (leakage when coughing or straining).

This table has some wildly large ranges, which reflects just how different the reported outcomes can be, study-to-study, hospital-to-hospital. In general, I would recommend ignoring the best and the worst results and using the middle values as more likely predictors of your outcome for each of the various treatments.[7,8,9,10,11]

3

Erectile Dysfunction after Prostate Cancer

YOUR PENIS AND ERECTIONS

By this point in your life, you undoubtedly are familiar with the two states of the penis: flaccid and erect. Most of the time, your penis is flaccid, not erect, which is normal. You are diagnosed with erectile dysfunction (ED) when your penis is never erect, or never hard enough for a long enough period of time for sexual gratification.

Recent developments in basic science and clinical research over the last 20 years or so have led to a better understanding of the mechanisms that regulate erectile function and treatments to help alleviate dysfunction. Learning about the basics of the penis and how it becomes erect will help you understand your condition, ask your doctor good questions, and make informed decisions about the various treatments available.

An Anatomy Lesson

The penis is one of several erectile organs in the human body. "Erectile" is an adjective meaning that they swell in size when more blood flows through them or is trapped in them. For example, the nipples of men and women and the labia, vagina, and clitoris of women swell with blood during sexual excitement. Even the lining of the nose has erectile tissue—cold medicines shrink this tissue to keep it from blocking your airway when you are congested.

To become erect, the penis depends on three sinus-like chambers collectively known as "the corporal bodies": the cylindrical *corpus spongiosum,* which runs down the underside of the penis, and two *corpora cavernosa,* which lie on either side of the corpus spongiosum (see Figure 3.1 below). The single *corpus spongiosum* (Latin for "body" and "sponge-like") holds the urethra, the tube where urine and semen pass. The corpus spongiosum is directly connected to the head or glans of the penis. The corpus spongiosum does not become rigid but during sexual excitement both the glans and the corpus spongiosum swell with extra blood.

The paired *corpora cavernosa* (Latin for "sinusoidal blood-filled chambers") are the two bodies responsible for the penis being either soft or erect. There is always some blood flowing in and out of these chambers (and the corpus spongiosum) to bring oxygen to the cells that make up the chambers. The usual rate of blood flow is about 10 milliliters per minute, or two teaspoons' full; for an erection, the penis needs extra blood to fill up the chambers. This is controlled via the relaxation of the smooth muscle cells that compose the cavernous bodies. Figure 3.2 shows the smooth muscle cells and corporal bodies of the penis. Smooth muscle is different from the muscles that control your arms or legs

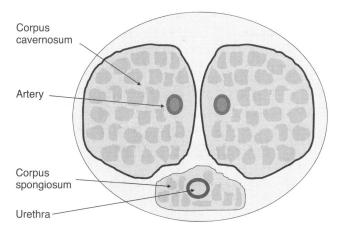

Figure 3.1 The relationship of the corporal bodies that allow penile erection. The two cavernous bodies become erectile. The corpus spongiosum swells with blood but remains soft.
(Courtesy of Kelvin Davies, PhD).

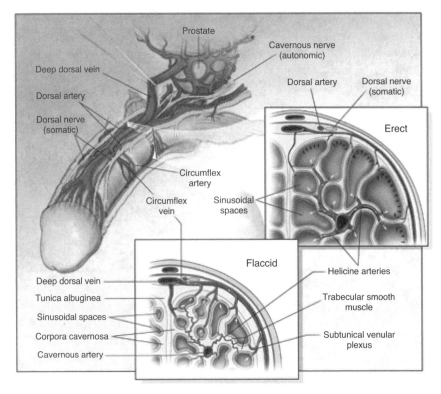

Figure 3.2 The anatomy of the penis in the flaccid and erect state. The difference is caused by blood filling the sinusoidal spaces of the corporal bodies. The blood is supplied by the cavernous artery that expands during sexual excitement. The relaxed smooth muscle cells that form the trabecular smooth muscle network prevent the blood from leaving the penis, and it remains erect until sexual excitement ceases.
(Reprinted with permission from the *New Eng J Med*. Copyright © 2000 Massachusetts Medical Society. All rights reserved.)

because unlike those muscles, you have no control over the smooth muscle fibers and cannot voluntarily contract or relax them.

When smooth muscle cells are relaxed, blood flows into the penis and is trapped in the cavernous bodies. When the muscles are contracted, they keep blood out of the penis, causing the penis to be flaccid.

Fluid Dynamics

The blood-trapping mechanism of the corporal bodies is critical for restricting blood outflow from the penis and maintaining an erection. Although the comparison may seem odd, this mechanism functions like the flap valve in a toilet tank. In a toilet, when the flap valve is down, no water escapes the tank. When the valve in the tank is raised, water leaves the tank and the toilet flushes.

Roughly, the same thing happens in the penis. (When these flaps don't work, it could be likened to toilet water continuously running after a flush. Unfortunately, fixing this problem isn't quite as easy as jiggling the handle.)

When a man is sexually aroused, his brain sends a signal to the tissues of the penis to relax; the flaps open and blood enters the corporal chambers. An erection forms when the penis fills with blood and the blood pressure within the penis is the same as the pressure in the arteries. This special valve-like network has a reproduction function: blood cannot be squeezed from the erect penis, a protective mechanism that keeps the strong squeezing muscles of a woman's vagina from making the penis soft during intercourse. After sex, the muscles within the penis tighten and the valve opens: blood is now free to drain from the penis.

The Brain Behind the Erection

Contrary to some claims, getting an erection also involves a man's brain—in fact, the whole central nervous system is involved. The hypothalamus, deep within the center of the brain, controls erections. The hypothalamus constantly suppresses an erection by sending electrical signals that travel down the nerves in the spinal cord, exit in the lower back, and pass through a collection of nerves, all the way to the penis. These signals essentially tell the penis to stay soft.

During sexual excitement–from visual, tactile, auditory, or psychological stimulation—other areas of the brain actively suppress the inhibitory signals from the hypothalamus and send their own signals down the spinal cord. These signals exit through nerves in the lower back and travel to the penis near the prostate gland, where they send signals to increase the flow of blood and make the penis erect.

You don't have to be consciously stimulated to get an erection. During a phase of sleep called rapid eye movement (REM), or dream sleep, excitatory signals are sent from the brain to the penis. This occurs four or five times a night, causing rigid erections that last about 15 minutes each. These are essentially workouts for your penis so that its structures remain in good health. During these REM erections, the penile chambers and cells receive extra oxygen and nutrients via the blood supply. The most intense of the REM erections usually occur just as you are about to wake up in the early morning (known in most college dorms as "morning wood"). REM erections occur in healthy men throughout life. Disease or old age, however, may cause these erections to be diminished in duration or frequency.

Interestingly, if the brain is not getting enough oxygen, the inhibitory signals may stop and an erection occurs. Some people deliberately trigger this type of erection by reducing their oxygen levels through "erotic asphyxiation," a dangerous sexual game that may cause or prolong an erection but may also lead to death by strangulation or suffocation (as it did for the actor David Carradine in 2009). Men executed by hanging sometimes die with an erection for the same reason.

Ejaculation

The ability to ejaculate, even for men who are past the child-bearing years, can be very important to the feeling of sexual satisfaction, so its loss should not be taken lightly. One report showed that 45% of the men who could not ejaculate after prostate surgery for non-cancerous disease felt that they had a deterioration of their sexual function.[1] There is no actual physical cause for this belief, but to these men, the loss of ejaculate alone seemed to adversely affect their sexual experience.

Ejaculate is made up of two basic components: sperm and seminal fluid. Only 1% of what you ejaculate is sperm; 99% is semen, made by two glands: the prostate and seminal vesicles. Seminal fluid contains nutrients and enzymes to keep sperm alive and mobile so that they can fertilize an egg.

Normal ejaculation happens in two steps. The first is the readying of emission: fluids from the seminal vesicles and prostate gland and sperm from the vas deferens are deposited into a holding in the prostatic urethra. This happens during the rhythmic contraction of smooth muscle in the walls of these organs as you near orgasm. The accumulation of this fluid precedes what people commonly refer to as ejaculation—projectile ejaculation of semen—by 1 or 2 seconds.

The ejaculation phase occurs with the simultaneous closure of the bladder neck and opening of the urinary sphincter and contraction of the muscles that surround the urethra. These actions together allow the propulsion of ejaculate. Orgasm, however, is a sensation apart from ejaculation and can still occur, even with damage to the nerves that control ejaculation. It will be an orgasm without ejaculation of the semen, or a "dry" orgasm, but the sensations can be just as pleasurable. This can be disconcerting at first, but all the great feelings of an orgasm will still be present.

When you start having sex again after surgery, you may initially have some pain in your lower abdomen when you orgasm; this is caused by the muscles of the pelvis contracting during orgasm and irritating some scar tissue in the surgical area. This does not mean that there is anything wrong from the surgery or that the cancer has returned. There is also a percentage of men who, after radical prostatectomy, expel small amounts of urine when they orgasm. Presumably urine leaks out from the bladder into the first part of the urethra and during the expulsion of ejaculation, the urine is forced out. If it is happening to you,

I suggest that you empty your bladder before having sex. There is no danger to your partner if it does happen.

HOW TO KNOW IF YOU HAVE A PROBLEM

Struggling with ED can be disheartening: A man tries to get hard, but the penis stays soft, or he gets erect but loses it quickly—all without ejaculation occurring. Some men report to their doctor that they have ED when they really mean that they lose their erection naturally after premature ejaculation (PE). After prostate cancer surgery, some men may have orgasm faster than they want and loose the erection prema-

> *"I was totally misled bout ED. About 30 or more days after surgery I got a semi-erection and was able to orgasm with effort. Around 90 days after surgery I started to get erections. I took pills (Viagra, Levitra) for three months or so; by March [5 months after surgery], I was off them and don't use them any more—kissing my wife does it for me."*
> *—Jake T., 59 years old at time of surgery*

turely, although there is no longer any ejaculate to expel. If you are unsure whether your problems need additional therapy, then read on.

Erectile Dysfunction after Surgery

After any major medical procedure, it takes the body about 6 weeks to get back to normal. During the first 6 weeks after any kind of treatment, you should take a break from sex and let your body recover. Of course, some patients recover faster and may want to "test the waters" after 4 or 5 weeks. You should be capable of feeling the desire to have sex and having an erection and orgasm—but no ejaculation—within about 40 days following surgery.

After surgery, your erections will improve naturally for up to 18 months post-op as the nerves that have been injured return to better function. During that time, your erections might not be hard enough for penetration or might not last long enough to be have successful intercourse. For those months, you might use temporary measures to improve erections such as the PDE5 inhibitors, intracavernous injections, or the vacuum erection device (*see* Chapter 4 for more information on these options). You will know whether you have a more lasting ED problem if 18 months have passed and your every effort to achieve erection is unsuccessful. At that point, you should pursue additional follow-up treatment, first with the urologist who did your surgery, then perhaps a sex therapist as well.

Erectile Dysfunction after Radiation

After radiation treatment, you may continue to have normal erections at first, then as time passes, you may lose the ability to obtain and maintain a satisfactory erection. This is because it takes time for the radiation to damage the necessary nerves. As above, you may use temporary measures at first, while continuing to periodically try to get erect without any aids. It usually takes 18 to 24 months for the body to bounce back after a bout of radiation, but every patient is different, depending on his pretreatment health and other medical problems. In any case, when you begin to feel it has been too long since your last "natural" erection, then it is time to go back to the doctor to be re-evaluated.

As discussed above, post-operative orgasms will be "dry" orgasms. What's less well-known is that radiation therapy can cause a decrease or absence of semen ejaculate as well: After brachytherapy, the reports vary from 7% to 45%; after external beam radiation therapy (EBRT), it ranges from 2% to 56%.[2]

REVIVING YOUR SEX-LIFE POST-TREATMENT

After completing cancer treatment, the first and normal response for most people is often relief that it's over and went well. Next, people often wonder: "Did the surgeon get all the cancer?" or "Did the radiation kill all the cancer cells?" It may take years to fully answer these questions. During this time, the stress can be a constant weight. This anxiety, by itself, can interfere with the ability to get an erection. If a man is in this situation, he may think just avoiding the issue is the right way to go. But depending on his age and relationship, years might pass before he gets the "all clear," or he may suffer a recurrence of the cancer. In either case, we encourage you (if you have a willing partner) to not let those months or years slip by without sex.

On the other hand, some men may rush prematurely into trying to have sex with their partners after the surgery. It is normal for a man who has been treated for prostate cancer to be anxious about whether or not he will be able to have erections. He may want to get back into "action" before his body is ready and can be disappointed when things don't work as desired. Low performance can occur *because* he is anxious and/or because the nerves that help control erections have not yet recovered their full function. It may take up to 18 months for any nerves injured during surgery or radiation to recover completely. Additionally, the anxiety may grow with each effort at sex, worsening the problem over time.

An important first step is to tell your doctor your concerns. If you simply answer "fine" when your doctor asks how things are going, he may never ask follow-up questions (although he should) to discover what's really going on.

Your doctor *should* ask you about your sexual function during your follow-up visits. Most people who have undergone prostate cancer treatment are willing and able to talk about this. However, if a patient says nothing, then it is likely a physician will not spend much time exploring the issue. In a busy office, doctors are always worried about the time they have available for each patient. Therefore, it is important for you to raise the subject even if your doctor does not. Don't let shyness or embarrassment stop you from getting the information you want. Recognize that this communication should be a two-way street;

Table 3.1. QUESTIONS TO ASK AT YOUR FIRST POST-TREATMENT DOCTOR'S VISIT:

- When can I resume having sex?
  I usually tell people to wait 6 weeks before resuming sex. By that time all of the wounds should be well-healed. The same goes for radiation—the tissue should be allowed to "calm down" after the radiation assault for approximately 6 weeks. All patients respond differently and if they recover faster and want to "test the waters," they can do so after 4 or 5 weeks.

- What can I expect in terms of sensation and feelings?
  A man's libido (sex drive) and ability to have orgasm can be normal or may be affected by the anxiety of cancer and its treatment. Skin sensation will be normal. The actual degree of erection is highly variable. Most men will be anxious about whether they will be able to have an erection and that, by itself, can create an erectile problem. Remember, after surgery, the erection will improve over the next 18 months. After radiation of any type, you might start just fine and then see your ability to get erections decline as the radiation enters the body, but it too should resolve after 18 to 24 months.

- How often should I try?
  Ideally, sex should be spontaneous and not a contrived event. Our recommendation is to have sex as often as you and your partner have the desire to do so. That being said, you may consider scheduling regular sex "dates" if your recovery is a slow one, just to ensure that you do not avoid the issue because the first few attempts didn't work out. It is important to keep trying because as your recovery progresses, your physical and emotional health will improve. Remember that "sex" comes in many flavors and may mean hugging, kissing, caressing, and oral sex, as well as intercourse.

- Will my partner notice a difference in sensation?
  There will be no changes in sensation with intercourse that your partner will perceive unless your erection is less rigid. If your partner has had children with vaginal delivery, her vagina may be relaxed enough to accept entry with a partial erection.

- Can I have children?
  Probably yes, but not the usual way. Keeping in mind that during a prostatectomy the tubes from the testes that carry sperm have been cut, it is not possible to conceive a child through intercourse because there is no ejaculate fluid. However, there is a new and technically possible procedure that "harvests" sperm directly from the testes to use for artificial insemination that can provide many safe and effective methods for conception.

- Are there any dos or don'ts in bed?
  Some men fear that they may pass on the cancer cells to their partner when they are having sex. That is not an issue with prostate cancer, and there is no risk to your partner at all if you have sex. Moreover, there are no restrictions in having sex following any treatment for prostate cancer, as there is no danger in making the tumor return or grow if you have sex. However, if you've had surgery, use caution in the first 6 weeks as the incision takes time to heal, even minimally invasive ones that are small. Aggravating the incision area can cause a hernia, no matter how small your incision was or what method of surgery was used.

- Should I be on a "pill support program?"
  The drug companies that manufacture Viagra, Cialis, and Levitra have supported studies showing that by taking a pill every day after surgery, there may be a greater chance of having a return to normal erections. However, in the largest study, in 628 men who were given either a placebo (sugar pill), nightly Levitra, or on-demand Levitra for 9 months, the results showed no difference between the groups.[a] Although there is experimental evidence in rats to show that PDE5 administration deceased penile scarring, there is no similar, secure evidence in man. Although the "pill support program" is in vogue, the scientific evidence is not secure enough to warrant the programs' cost—both in dollars and in dashed hopes. It may be that the pills allow the cells of the penis to stay healthier during the recovery from the surgery, thus allowing erections to return. However, more research is needed from more objective investigators to verify these first results.

- What are the non-medical options for dealing with ED?
  The only FDA-approved non-medical aid that has been advocated is the vacuum erection device (VED). That device is described more fully in Chapter 4 on page 76. There have been only a few clinical trials with this device in men following radical prostatectomy. In one study the men who used the VED had a lower return of erections than those who did not use it (32% vs. 37 %.)[b] In another small study of 28 men, 17 of whom used the VED daily for two 5-minute sessions, the return of normal erectile function (although better than the control group who did not use the VED) was minimal and did not return the men to normal, spontaneous erections.[c]

- What are alternatives to medication to assist in recovery to sexual health?
  If your doctor is more interested in discussing the outcomes of the surgery or radiation therapy than in some of the side effects or complications of the treatment, ask politely (but insist) on the name of and referral to someone who is a specialist in sexual health and erectile function. If more than one person is recommended, interview them either in person or, more practically, over the phone to decide who is the best fit for you. It is difficult to feel absolutely comfortable talking about the most intimate details of your sex life, but the right doctor will help you and your partner to feel okay (keep in mind you may never feel completely comfortable, but it will be worth the effort to do so). Your partner will definitely be involved if you go to a sex therapist, and if you choose a urologist, your partner should accompany you on at least the first visit but should be welcome at any and every appointment. (See Chapter 4 for a detailed list of ED treatments—there's more to this than Viagra, which does not work on all men.)

[a] Montorsi et al., (2008) *European Urol* 54:924–931.
[b] Raina et al., (2006) *Int J Imp Res* 18:77–81.
[c] Kohler et al., (2007) *BJU Int* 100:858–862.

you need to offer him or her honest information about your body so that your doctor can best assess your situation and advise you on solving the problem.

ERECTILE DYSFUNCTION ISSUES AND SURGERY

The primary cause of severe ED after surgery is nerve damage that occurs during the operation. However, that is not the only factor that determines which patients return to normal erectile function. If you do develop ED after surgery, there are several good treatment options that can enable you to regain your sex life.

Nerve-Sparing Surgery

Even when the best "nerve-sparing" prostatectomy is performed by the most skilled surgeon, there can sometimes be a reduction in nerve function. There are several types of surgeries for treating prostate cancer, including radical retropubic prostatectomy, laparoscopic retropubic prostatectomy, robotic retropubic prostatectomy, and radical perineal prostatectomy. Your surgeon will use the approach with which he or she has the most experience and that is best suited to your situation. (*See* Chapter 2 for descriptions of these approaches.)

Most prostate cancer surgeons try to spare both the right and left sets of nerves that control erection. These nerves travel alongside and over the outer surface of the prostate. Some of these nerves also enter the prostate while the rest run into the surface of the urethra. Very few of these tiny nerves actually enter erectile tissue of the penis.

The decision to spare both sets of nerves is usually made based on the size of the cancer, where the cancer is located, and whether the surgeon believes that the tumor has spread outside the covering of the prostate. Most surgeons will not attempt nerve-sparing surgery if cancer extends outside the prostate's surface. The first priority of any doctor in this situation is to save the patient's life through effective removal of the cancer.

In an ideal world—where the cancer is localized and the surgeon has a high degree of expertise—bilateral (both sides) nerve sparing via robotic surgery often offers the best chance of a return to sexual function. There are several reasons for this. Robotic surgery is done with the use of a gas to push aside the abdominal organs, which allows a good view of the surgical site. The gas limits bleeding, also improving the view of the surgery site. Additionally, the operative field is magnified by the lenses and the television camera, giving very clear, three-dimensional views of the prostate for the surgeon. Because nerves can be difficult to see and easy to bump against, anything that gives the surgeon a clearer view of the area is an advantage in successful nerve sparing.

Radical perineal prostatectomy would be next in line in terms of best surgical field view and ease of surgery. Next would be laparoscopic surgery followed by the radical retropubic.

Remember there are still other factors to consider in choosing a surgery. Where is your cancer? What is the size of your prostate? And, of course, what is the surgeon's experience? A surgeon who has done 10 robotic surgeries versus someone who has performed a thousand radical retropubic operations is less likely to have the same outcome of good nerve sparing. Before you choose a surgeon, make sure you ask about his or her surgical experience and preferences.

Other Factors that Determine Erectile Function Recovery

If you had a bilateral (both sides) nerve-sparing operation, you have the best chance for complete recovery of erectile function. The chance of your recovery depends on your age, the amount of sexual activity you had before surgery, the quality of your erection before the operation, your other illnesses, and medications you take. If both sets of nerves were destroyed, then there is little chance of your erection returning. If only one side was destroyed, then you have a better chance for the return of an erection.

As a general guide, a man in his early 50s with no other illnesses and a small cancer should have a better expected outcome and return to a near normal sexual

---

A PATIENT'S STORY: ERECTILE DYSFUNCTION AFTER SURGERY

Edward B. was only in his 50s when a routine blood test showed an elevated PSA; a biopsy soon revealed he had prostate cancer. He immediately set to work researching treatments and was still weighing his options when his friends intervened, urging him to hurry up and "get it out of there!" He had surgery, which seemed to have worked on the cancer, although it left him dealing with both ED and urinary incontinence. However, a few years later, Edward's PSA rose again. This time he was put on Lupron (hormone suppression) therapy. The Lupron kept his PSA at 0 for a decade or so, despite unpleasant side effects. "It gave me tits," he deadpanned, "I'm an A-minus!" Fast forward a couple of years, Edward had met a steady partner and wanted to regain his sex life. He tried everything—Viagra didn't help, and the injections were more trouble than he wanted. Eventually, he opted for a penile implant, the "gooseneck lamp" kind. "I was glad I had it done," he stated. Today he is 76 years old and has lived more than 25 fruitful years since his diagnosis.

---

life than a 65-year-old man with obesity, diabetes, and hypertension who was already noticing a decline in his ability to have prolonged and rigid erections. If you enjoyed a thriving sex life with a loving, understanding partner before treatment, then you will probably have an easier time than if you rarely had sex pre-cancer and do not have a strong relationship that can withstand a little experimentation. That said, everybody's experience is different and needs to be evaluated individually by a physician. It is especially unwise to compare your situation with research study results you find on the internet. The researchers and clinicians writing the report may pick and choose their study candidates (e.g., only younger men) and give unrealistic results or expectations for a post-operative return to erections. Rather than getting upset by comparing yourself to other people, talk to your surgeon before and after the surgery about your chances for regaining satisfying erections.

ERECTILE DYSFUNCTION AND RADIATION TREATMENT

After receiving radiation treatment, men may think that at first, everything is okay, but sometimes they begin to lose erectile function little by little, in the weeks and months after treatment. Unlike surgery, where the injury to the nerves happens immediately, damage to the nerves from radiation occurs over time and in fact worsens over the course of treatment and post-treatment time. It usually takes 18 to 24 months for the radiation effects to wear off. Radiation affects the nerves, blood vessels, and the tissues at the base of the penis. The resulting changes on those structures vary, from little to total, and are affected by the age and sexual activity before therapy. Men who are younger (less than 60 years of age) and who have normal erectile function before treatment will be less affected by the radiation than older men who already have some deterioration of function. It is normal for all men as they age to have a reduction in erectile function. If ED symptoms persist over a 3-month period, then a man should follow up with his medical team to determine whether other treatments can to be used to accomplish intercourse.

Radiation is a high-energy beam that kills cells by making them die a premature death or by preventing them from dividing. The goal is to only kill cancer cells, but inevitably healthy cells are also destroyed. Some cancers are killed with very low doses of radiation (e.g., seminoma, a form of testicular cancer) but prostate cancer is resistant to radiation and often needs high doses of energy for treatment. The radiation therapists go to great length to minimize the effect of radiation on non-cancer cells, but sometimes even the best efforts cannot prevent some damage from occurring. There are two common ways that radiation therapy is delivered. External beam radiation therapy uses a machine that aims X-rays at the body. Brachytherapy places one of two types of radioactive seeds into the prostate. (*See* Chapter 2 for an in-depth explanation of these approaches.) Some patients who have large prostate glands, a more aggressive tumor, or a tumor that is close to the edge of the prostate may receive both seeds and EBRT.

Radiation can be delivered specifically to the prostate gland (called *prostate-only radiation*) or also encompass the surrounding pelvic lymph nodes (called *whole pelvic radiation*). Evaluating the pelvis and surrounding area tells the doctor whether the entire prostate and the nodes in the prostate area are all targeted for treatment. Whether through EBRT, or brachytherapy, the radiation from within can still affect the same nerves.

A PATIENT'S STORY: ERECTILE DYSFUNCTION AFTER RADIATION

When Michael K. was diagnosed with prostate cancer in his early 70s, he was "surprised, but I felt confident about the treatment." Because of a heart condition, Michael was not a good surgery candidate, so his doctor prescribed 39 treatments of EBRT. He didn't have any problems during treatment but did several months later: mainly erectile dysfunction, which never improved. He did not pursue other treatments for ED because of his heart condition—he had open-heart surgery and took nitroglycerin, which meant no Viagra. "I was not happy about it, by then I was about 72 years old, but that's the way it developed." Today, Michael is 90 years old and about to celebrate his 60th wedding anniversary. He has beaten cancer again—this time of the larynx—and is dealing with both diabetes and congestive heart failure. "My prostate cancer woes pale in comparison," he says. "But I'm basically an optimist. I don't let it deject me or anything. Attitude is very important."

PSYCHOLOGICAL ASPECTS OF ERECTILE DYSFUNCTION

In Chapter 9, we will discuss the psychological issues related to prostate cancer recovery, but it is important to mention here how critical your mental health is to healthy erectile function. As noted earlier in this chapter, the entire central nervous system co-operates in the production of an erection. Psychological problems can disrupt that intricate cooperative system and cause ED in an otherwise physically healthy person. Anxiety, loss of confidence, and depression are relatively frequent psychological problems that can follow prostate cancer treatment and limit the return to a healthy sex life. Among the issues particular to prostate cancer patients may be the fear of:

- Having cancer
- Major surgery
- No longer "being a man" after the surgery
- Erectile dysfunction
- Urinary incontinence
- Recurrence of the cancer
- Fear of death and aging
- Accompanying anxiety or depression from any of the above fears.

A PATIENT'S STORY: TRYING TOO HARD

John S.'s PSA had been in the normal range for a man his age (62 years) but, after a sudden jump in the PSA number from one year to the next, he had a biopsy. His clinical diagnosis was a prostate-confined, Gleason's grade 6 tumor. He chose to undergo a robotic nerve-sparing radical prostatectomy.

His sex life was fine before surgery and his only medicine was for hypertension. His surgeon had told him he had a 90% chance of having normal erections after surgery. By the third month after his operation, he was trying every day to have sex with his wife but could not develop any penile rigidity.

The doctor was puzzled, because the patient had said that 8 weeks after surgery he had begun to again have early morning erections that were hard enough to have sex. But the more times John and his wife tried to have sexual intercourse, the worse his ED became. He got extremely frustrated and disappointed, was on the verge of depression, and doubted his treatment decisions.

The return of morning erections and an excellent health and sex history suggested that John should have had a full recovery. As his doctor explained to him, he needed to stop trying so hard. One suggestion was to be sexual with his partner without coitus as a goal; this often decreases "penetration pressure." Not trying so frequently would also be helpful. There were also some medical interventions that could be helpful for John in the interim. A medication such as Levitra, Viagra, or Cialis or small doses of intracavernous therapy would probably be helpful to John as he got his confidence back.

It worked! After some successful medically induced erections, John's performance anxiety slowly decreased and he returned to normal erectile function.

It is critical and helpful that you receive repetitive reassurance from your doctor addressing the above fears. If you are not getting the support you need from your doctor, then you have some choices: you could bring up the subject to your doctor and pursue the care you seek; you could try talking to your primary care doctor or another trusted member of your medical care team (sometimes nurse practitioners or physicians' assistants have more time than MDs for a quiet talk); you could ask for a referral to a psychologist or psychiatrist; you could content yourself with confiding in friends and family; or you could find a support group in your area for cancer patients—prostate cancer is not the only cancer whose treatment leads to anxiety and sexual dysfunction. Time also plays a significant role. One of the great truisms in medicine is that time heals many ailments. Sexual function and enjoyment often returns as the weeks and months pass from the time of surgery and the man sees that he is well, the cancer has not returned, he no longer has problems with urinary leakage, and his sexual partner has not left him.

It is hard to differentiate psychological from physical causes of ED, especially for men who worry a lot about the problem, because the more they worry, the more anxious they become and, in turn, the problem worsens. I usually suggest they visit a professional who deals with sexual problems. Urologists, particularly those who specialize in male sexual dysfunction, can best make the correct assessment of whether it is a physical or psychological problem. In the next chapter, we'll address the treatments for ED of any cause.

Treatments for Erectile Dysfunction

By their late teens, most men already take their erections for granted—whenever they need one, it is there. For the next two or three decades, the idea that erections are always "easy" and physically spontaneous is further cemented by years of regular sexual activity, alone and/or with partners. But around age 50 years, the problems that most affect erectile function, such as hypertension and atherosclerosis (hardening of the arteries), diabetes, high blood pressure medication, and aging (which on its own causes erectile problems), begin to arrive. Some men begin to lose their easy erectile function around this time as a result of these factors; others continue to have good erections up into their 70s. Prostate cancer treatment can put an end to that. Indeed, almost every treatment will cause at least a temporary case of erectile dysfunction (ED).

Sex with a quick, rigid erection is usually the kind of sex we are used to having, the kind of sex we discuss with friends and lovers, the kind of sex we watch in movies and TV. It is so rare to see or hear of other types of sex—sex with erections that take more time or involve a little planning—that we usually forget that there *is* any other kind of sex. Even if we know not all erections are rock hard and instantaneous, we are still convinced that is the only kind of erection worth having. Perhaps you feel that sex without a quick erection isn't worth the trouble. For a while after treatment, you may feel like there is nothing left of your sexual life, but remember that even when you develop ED, the other phases of male sexuality—libido, orgasm, and ejaculation—may continue to function normally. A pleasurable, fulfilling sexual life can continue for you, but it is one that probably includes less spontaneity and requires more effort from both partners. It is important (and difficult) to embrace the idea that *a changed sex life can still be a good sex life.* You and your partner may take this leap of faith together, or you may be taking it alone. Either way, know that many other men have traveled this path before you, and there can be years of satisfying sex ahead.

With all that said, patients with ED after prostate cancer treatment are usually very disheartened by the problem; even when warned in advance of the possibility, most think that it will not happen to them. After treatment, they realize that it *can* happen to them and they are not happy about it. In particular, younger men who have had an active sex life pre-therapy are usually angry and depressed. Their wives and significant others may be as well, putting further pressure on the man to perform sexually. After any of the therapies, I remind patients that the principal goal of the therapy is *to cure the cancer.* A doctor who administers less than adequate treatment in order to preserve a patient's potency does not do that patient any favors—and that will become clear when the cancer recurs or spreads. I often remind patients that a dead man cannot have sex, but a living man with ED and cured cancer can be helped in many ways to resume his sexual life. That is the focus of this chapter.

As noted in Chapter 3, even if prostate cancer treatment goes well and is administered by the best doctors in the best hospitals, nearly every type of treatment can leave the patient with at least a temporary case of ED.

There are several different causes of ED for post-prostate cancer patients. Damage to the nerves and blood vessels that feed the extra blood into the penis and are needed to maintain the normal erectile response during surgery and radiation can also cause ED. Similarly, prevalent causes are normal psychological responses to the stress of having cancer and recovering from treatment. See Chapter 3 for a complete discussion of how different treatments can trigger ED.

PSYCHOLOGICAL RESPONSES TO PROSTATE CANCER AS ERECTILE DYSFUNCTION TRIGGERS

It is important to separate psychologically triggered ED from ED rooted in physical problems, because psychological ED is the only type of ED that is 100% curable. (With most physical ED, some kind of ongoing treatment is usually necessary to resume your sex life.) We say this not to scare you, but to give you hope: you don't have to live with ED or give up sex! There are solutions to the problem, especially if it started in your head.

Some men's erectile problems are a result not of physical side effects but of the psychological toll of prostate cancer and its treatment. Among the most common responses to any cancer diagnosis are fear, anxiety, and depression. With prostate cancer, there are specific fears that hit men where it hurts: fears of ED, of incontinence, of being "less of a man," or being unable to please your partner.

These fears are completely normal and should not be minimized by the patient himself, his doctor, his partner, or his friends and family. Every patient will probably experience such feelings to a degree, but some patients can develop ED from these fears, even if their physical anatomy is still fully capable of erections.

To determine whether it is your feelings that are getting in the way of your "sexual healing" or some other cause, your doctor can prescribe a nighttime erection test. That test, developed in the 1980s, is called nocturnal penile tumescence testing. A device called the Rigiscan measures the number, duration, and hardness of erections while you sleep. It is a computer-based instrument made for use in the privacy of your home. During the rapid eye movement (REM) period of sleep, men normally have four or five 15- to 20-minute erections. The Rigiscan has a component that wraps around the penis, measures the erections, and downloads the results to a computer that can provide a printout for your physician.

The best REM erection occurs in the early morning. If you have that early morning erection after your treatment, it means that you are physically capable of having an erection for sex as well. You can also ask your willing wife or partner to observe you during the night to see if you get erections. Be forewarned that depression and sleep disorders such as sleep apnea can limit time spent in REM sleep, which can affect the test's outcome—the test might give a false result, implying that you cannot get normal erections when you really can. There is not much to do about that except to interpret the test with caution and repeat it at a later date when things may have changed (e.g., after treating or ruling out any apnea or depression).

Psychologically triggered ED in patients with otherwise-normal erectile function causes the same problems when the man has ED that arises solely from physical problems: The man tries to get hard, but the penis stays soft, or he gets erect but loses it quickly and is unable to sustain his erection to have intercourse. If severe depression or anxiety is the cause, he may even lose all desire to have sex. In either case, it is important to treat the physical effects of ED as well as the root psychological causes of the problem.

How to Treat Psychological Erectile Dysfunction

If it is determined that your ED is not a physically rooted problem, it can be helpful to get a referral from your treating physician to an individual or couples therapist to help work through any fears or anxieties in a safe, nonjudgmental environment. Going to a therapist does not mean you are crazy. Look at it this way: if you had a rash on your skin that you wanted to clear up, then you would go to a dermatologist; if you had prostate cancer, then you would go to a urologist or oncologist. Psychologists and psychiatrists can help you "clear up" problems that are emotional—and everyone, whether a cancer patient or not, has some emotional problems that could use clearing up. Therapists are trained to be good listeners and to help you make sense of your new reality. Many men also find improvement in their mental state simply by sharing their own experiences, with a spouse, friend (often one has survived similar trials is a good choice), or even anonymously in prostate cancer Internet "chat rooms." (Some recommended internet and other resources are listed in the Appendix.)

Until the invention of certain medical-grade silicone polymers in the 1960s, the bulk of the treatment for *any* ED was psychological therapy. This treatment did not help a man whose ED had a *physical* cause very much, but talking to a third sympathetic party probably allayed some of the anxiety that comes with any case of ED. Psychological therapy for anxiety and depression is always an appropriate treatment for those problems. In my experience, men who have appropriate insurance coverage or funding are willing to go for such therapy. However, the therapists have traditionally been less frequently covered by insurance (although now that mental health parity was recently instituted by the Federal government, that should no longer be true) and are not always available in rural areas, so it frequently has become the province of the family physician or urologist to do what they can. In Chapters 9 and 10, we will discuss the psychological aspects of recovery in depth, including the use of the internet as an alternative means of couples therapy that can bypass availability and financial issues.

A successful adjunct treatment for psychological ED, along with sex or psychological therapy, could be medication that would allow erections (such as Viagra) but not cure the primary depression or anxiety. Sometimes a temporary medical intervention helps a man regain his confidence and eventually allows the anxiety to subside.

MEDICAL TREATMENTS FOR ERECTILE DYSFUNCTION

Easy medicinal treatment for most types of ED began with the invention of the "phosphodiesterase (PDE)-5 inhibitor" drugs: Viagra, Levitra, and Cialis.

They were not the first medical therapy for ED but are clearly the most successful. Their importance warrants a full discussion.

In addition to PDE-5 inhibitor pills, there are several other methods of administering erection-inducing drugs: intracavernous injections or direct insertion (commonly known as Muse). In the last two sections of this chapter, we will discuss a mechanical treatment (vacuum device) and permanent, surgical options (penile implants).

Treating Erectile Dysfunction with Phosphodiesterase-5 Inhibitors

Viagra, the first of the PDE-5 inhibitors, was introduced in 1996 and revolutionized ED treatment in many ways. For one thing, Viagra was the first proven treatment for ED that could be taken in oral form. From infancy on, we rely on taking treatments by mouth, whether antibiotics or aspirins, to make us feel better or satisfy our discomfort. The other treatments described below can be more effective than Viagra (depending on the man and the cause of his ED) but are more invasive than taking a pill, and this invasiveness turns off many men who could otherwise be helped.

The desire for a "magic ED pill" has been so strong that shysters have been exploiting it for years. One example is the drug Yohimbine, made from the bark of an African tree, which has been marketed successfully to treat ED, despite complete lack of scientific evidence that it is effective and no mention of side effects such as raising blood pressure or causing a stroke if too much is taken. Many worthless drugs or supplements made with exciting ingredients like "Horny Goatweed" are featured in ads that promise to remake every ED sufferer into a stud surrounded by gorgeous women. The consumer should not be conned by such advertising—such products enrich their makers but cannot remake you. Unlike those unproven oral remedies, PDE-5 inhibitors really can provide a "magic bullet" for some men with ED. But buyers beware: it does not work on every patient, nor will it guarantee that you will be surrounded with gorgeous young women.

> In the Sanskrit language, the word "viagra" means "tiger." Some might say that by taking the little blue pill, you are literally putting a tiger in your tank.

A second significant achievement of PDE-5 inhibitors is that the publicity accompanying the launch of these drugs has lessened the stigma of erectile dysfunction. Presidential candidates and famous athletes proudly announced (for money) that they had ED and took Viagra. Men with ED saw that they were not alone and saw that confident, successful men could have this problem, talk about it, and be helped. The continual advertising of PDE-5 inhibitors makes it less embarrassing to talk about, but it can also put pressure on men who are not able to perform sexually even if they take the pill. Generally, however, Viagra and similar drugs have managed to increase communication about the problem of ED and decrease the shame and stigma.

THE DISCOVERY OF PHOSPHODIESTERASE-5 INHIBITORS

Several decades ago, researchers at the pharmaceutical company Pfizer were testing a pill to treat heart problems when they noticed an interesting side effect. Men taking the experimental drug found their erections were much improved and did not want to stop taking the pills! The company quickly redesigned its research study to focus on this effect of the drug.

About 10 years earlier in Paris (1982), a vascular surgeon named Ronald Virag made a similar discovery. At the time, there was only one successful therapy for physical ED: penile prosthetic implants (fully described later in this chapter). During a routine diagnostic procedure, Dr. Virag was infusing saline into a patient's penis, not knowing that his nurse had accidentally included a drug, papaverine, in the solution. Papaverine is a drug routinely used by vascular surgeons to dilate (relax) blood vessels. When Virag injected the solution, the man immediately got an erection. Virag realized that by causing an erection without sexual stimulation through an injection of papaverine, he had come upon both a new potential treatment for ED and a new understanding of the true mechanism of erection. Prior to that time, it was not really understood that men get erections because of relaxation of the smooth muscle cells of the corpora cavernosal bodies and the arteries that feed the penis.

HOW THEY WORK

The drug Dr. Virag accidentally shot into his patient, papaverine, belongs to a family of drugs known as PDE inhibitors. Predominantly found in the male genitalia, PDE-5s are enzymes whose main job is preventing normal erections from going on forever. When a healthy man gets aroused, his brain signals pro-duction of a natural chemical that causes the smooth muscles in the penis to relax (the chemical is called cyclic guanosine monophosphate—thankfully nicknamed cGMP).

As detailed on page 46, the relaxation of smooth muscles allows the penis to get fully erect. The PDE-5 enzymes are like little Pac Men that eat up this erec-tion-causing cGMP. When the arousal reaction is in full swing, however, there is too much cGMP flooding into the genitals for the PDE-5s to keep up; the resulting glut of cGMP allows an erection to occur. After orgasm, the brain sends a signal to turn down the cGMP production and the PDE-5 Pac Men can easily eat up all cGMP. When the cGMP is all "eaten up," the smooth muscle cells of the penis stops relaxing, and the erection goes away.

In many men with ED, something disrupts the natural production of cGMP during arousal and what little cGMP is produced is easily eaten up by the PDE-5 enzymes. The PDE-5 inhibitor pills, such as Viagra, come to the rescue by blocking the PDE-5 Pac Men, which allows the amount of cGMP to grow unchecked. More cGMP means smooth muscle relaxation and better erections. Only when the drug wears off (a few hours later) do the PDE-5 Pac Men come back on duty and gobble up the cGMP, causing the erection to go down. (Figure 4.1 illustrates how PDE-5 inhibitors works.)

The PDE-5 inhibitors must be taken on demand, at least 30 to 60 minutes before the desired sexual act. Viagra must be taken on an empty stomach (at least two hours after eating). Levitra and Cialis can be taken after eating. The full effect of Viagra and Levitra lasts for about 8 hours. Cialis gives you a little more spontaneity because its duration is about a day and a half.

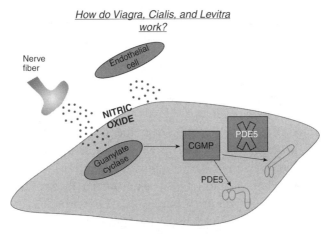

Figure 4.1 A conceptual drawing of how Viagra, Cialis, and Levitra cause erections. The gas nitric oxide (NO) is released from nerve endings and the cells that line the penis. The gas diffuses into the smooth muscle cells of the penile corpora and in turn activates the enzyme guanylate cyclase. The activated guanylate cyclase enzyme causes the production of cGMP, a chemical whose actions in the cell result in penile erection. The naturally occurring (in the smooth muscle cell) phosphodiesterase enzymes cause the destruction of cGMP to allow the penis to return to the non-erect state. Viagra, Cialis, and Levitra block the natural PDE enzyme and allow the penis to continue to be erect. When the NO is not released because the sexual signal stops, cGMP is not produced and the erection subsides, even in the presence of the Viagra, Cialis, and Levitra.

A new concept for treating prostate cancer patients with PDE-5 drugs has been to use daily or on-demand doses of these pills as a form of penile rehabilitation after radical prostatectomy. The theory behind the treatment is that daily, low doses of the drugs will in some way prevent or limit the smooth muscle damage that can be caused by nerve damage during a radical prostatectomy. Although the desired changes in the smooth muscle tissue have been found in animal studies, the results of two human studies have not shown similar results. At this time, the use of long-term penile rehabilitation with PDE-5 drugs is controversial and unproven.

SIDE EFFECTS AND RISKS

After you take a pill by mouth, it dissolves in your stomach and is absorbed in the small intestine. The drug then is taken into the bloodstream, traveling around to every organ in your body to exert its effect. The PDE-5 inhibitors don't know that they are being taken to cause an effect only on the penis to cause erections. So the drugs work in every organ that contains PDE-5 enzymes—remember we said most of them live in the genitalia, but not all! They can also be found in the face and scalp, the stomach and intestines, and the blood vessels of the brain—even the erectile tissue of the nose. The effect on all of these areas is the same: it prolongs the effect of cGMP and makes the smooth muscle cells relax. That may be what you want in your penis, but in the brain it can cause headaches; in the nose, nasal stuffiness; in the face, flushing. It can also cause vision abnormalities—some men describe "blue views" (a blue tinge to their vision) when taking these drugs.

PDE-5 inhibitors can also cause dilation and a drop in blood pressure, particularly if taken with alcohol or in the presence of blood pressure medications, especially the class of drugs known as alpha-blockers. If you are taking blood pressure-lowering pills, ask the doctor who prescribed them to you whether you are at risk when taking them with the PDE-5 inhibitors. The risks are important in most men, but especially in older men with low blood pressure or very high blood pressure and especially in men who use nitroglycerin products. Such men should absolutely avoid PDE-5 inhibitors.

The most serious risk of the PDE-5 inhibitors is in the men who use nitroglycerin products. The PDE-5 inhibitors can make these men lose consciousness or go into shock and can even cause death, because taking those drugs raises the level of cGMP in your blood, making the blood vessels around the body relax and causing a precipitous drop in blood pressure. Again, we stress that *men who take (or who may need to take) nitroglycerin and similar drugs (ask your doctor if you are unsure) absolutely must not take PDE-5 inhibitors.*

A very rare risk of PDE-5 inhibitors is a type of blindness called non-arteritic anterior ischemic optic neuropathy (NAION). This side effect occurs suddenly, upon awakening, with poor vision (a dark shadow) in one eye, involving the upper or lower half of vision. There is an increased risk of NAION in men with an abnormally shaped optic disc (diagnosed by your eye doctor) and in white men older than age 50 years with diabetes, increased blood pressure, coronary artery disease, increased fat in the blood, and history of smoking and/or heart attacks. The treatment for NAION is high doses of steroids given within two weeks of onset, with improvement in vision in occurring in about 70% of men compared to only 40% who were not treated within six months of the attack.

Another rare risk associated with the use of the PDE-5 inhibitors is sudden hearing loss– which has happened enough to warrant the FDA to require a warning of possible deafness must be included in the pills' labels. In nearly all cases the deafness occurs in only one ear and is permanent in two-thirds of cases.

A comparison of the side effects published by the three manufacturers, minus the placebo effect, is shown in Table 4.1.[1]

Why These Drugs May Succeed or Fail

Overall, PDE-5 inhibitors work in about 60% of the patients who try them. The PDE-5 inhibitors work best in men who are relatively healthy. They do not work well in men who have diabetes or low testosterone levels or in men who have nerve damage after a radical prostatectomy.

Because half of men with diabetes have ED, and so many men are diabetic, those men form a large proportion of men who need treatment. The reasons why the PDE-5 inhibitors do not work in those circumstances relates to the anatomy and functional structure of the penis. In diabetics, the tone of the smooth muscle cells is higher to begin with, meaning it is harder for diabetics' smooth muscles to relax, and the effect of cGMP caused by the PDE-5 inhibitors may not be enough to create and prolong erection.

Table 4.1. Side Effects of PDE-5 Inhibitors

Side effect	Viagra 25–100 mg	Levitra 5–20 mg	Cialis 20 mg
Headache	12%	11%	10%
Flushing	12%	10%	2%
Gastric distress	5% (17% at 100 mg)	3%	9%
Nasal congestion, sinusitis	2%	8%	2%
Dizziness	1%	1%	Not reported
Abnormal vision	11% at 100 mg	Not reported	Not reported
Back or muscle pain	0%	0.3%	5%

A Patient's Story: PDE-5 Inhibitor Use During Recovery

Mike N. is a 55-year-old married, sexually active man with a localized prostate cancer (Gleason's 7, PSA 3.7). He was in otherwise perfect health and took no medications before his cancer diagnosis. He underwent a nerve-sparing radical retropubic prostatectomy, and his post-operative PSA at 1 month after surgery was undetectable. He regained complete urinary control 5 weeks after the surgery and after that happened, he and his wife wanted to try to resume intercourse. He noted that he had partial erections when he awoke in the morning but they were not sufficiently hard for vaginal penetration. He was offered a PDE-5 inhibitor drug, and he elected to try the 20-mg dose of Cialis. The couple resumed intercourse, and over a period of 2 months, the erections, with the medication, were rigid. After 8 months he began trying to have sex without taking the drug, and by 1 year he had normal erections without any medication.

For Mike, the PDE-5 inhibitor got him through the time when his body and mind were still recovering from the cancer and surgery. The fact that he was able to recover normal erections after a year proved that his surgery had successfully spared the important nerves. However, that year might have been a long and difficult wait without the Cialis—Mike and his wife might have given up on their sex life, or had other complications in their relationship. Luckily, Mike took advantage of a little medical assistance until his own recovery was complete.

Low blood testosterone is another problem that makes PDE-5 inhibitors less effective. The mechanism is not completely understood but may be related to the effect that testosterone has on the smooth muscle cells in the penis. It seems that when the level of the blood testosterone is low, it is harder for the cells to relax. Until the hormonal problem is corrected, the PDE-5 inhibitors do not have enough effect to correct the ED problem. Low blood testosterone is a particular issue for men with prostate cancer because lowering the level of testosterone in the blood is used as therapy for men who do not have localized disease (either as a primary treatment or after surgery or radiation if the cancer recurs) and for some men who are having radiation therapy. Luckily, there are other treatments that may work for these men who are not helped by PDE-5 inhibitors. Low testosterone levels also lead to a lower sex drive, which can further challenge ED treatment for this population.

The final population not well-served by Viagra-like drugs are men who have nerves in the penile region damaged during prostate cancer surgery. After a radical prostatectomy, nerve damage may prevent the brain from signaling for cGMP, the chemical that causes smooth muscle relaxation. The PDE-5 inhibitors are not effective in these cases because cGMP is not being produced and therefore the PDE-5 Pac Men have nothing to eat; thus, inhibiting PDE-5s will not cause an erection.

So who are the patients for whom PDE-5 inhibitors work best? These are generally young-ish men who have few other health problems and men who are wealthy or well-insured. The cost of the Viagra, Levitra, and Cialis is a major issue in the United States. Out-of-pocket costs average $22 to $28 per pill. Most insurance companies, in an effort to maintain their profitability, will not pay for more than four pills per month in most cases and demand that your physician produce evidence to show that there is a physical and not a psychological cause of the ED. Other insurance companies claim that sex is not "medically necessary," and will not pay for any pills at all. To save money, some men order "real" Viagra from countries like India or China at a fraction of the price. Again, buyer beware: these drugs are not subject to the same quality control as drugs sold in North America and may not contain the right amount (or even the right drug) to cause the desired effect. Read on for more cost-efficient methods (or how to get more, ahem, bang for your bucks).

Intracavernous Injections

Intracavernous injections (ICI) are another method of solving ED through drug therapy. These injections work very well in men who have had radical prostate surgery, since the drugs bypass the erection-causing nerves that might be damaged in surgery. You would be referred to an urologist for this treatment, which involves injecting an erection-stimulating drug directly into the penis. If you can get past the combination of the words "injecting" and "penis," then there is much to recommend this therapy, which often proves effective when nothing else works. Unlike the PDE-5 inhibitor pills, it will make the man have an erection even if he is not sexually excited. One patient's wife commented that ICI "could give a dead man doing his taxes an erection."

There are three or four different drugs that can be used in these injections, which are first given in a doctor's office to test their effectiveness and whether the man is willing and able to use ICI on his own. Most urologists prescribe either a single drug (prostaglandin), or a combination of three drugs—prostaglandin, papaverine (the drug that started it all), and phentolamine. The injection is made in the side of the penis with a very small needle and in very small quantities because it is so effective. Most men say there is not much pain—just a quick pinprick—as the needle is very small and the shot is fast. The hardness and duration of the erection depends on the man's blood flow and the normalcy of the smooth muscles of the penis. Therefore, the dose of medicine that is needed is different for every man and must be individually determined by an experienced physician.

Usually the patients who choose this treatment have tried the PDE-5 inhibitors and Muse (*see* page 75) without success and now they have a choice of staying "as is," trying injections, or jumping to a penile prosthetic implant. ICI has about an 85% success rate. However, despite that high rate of success, the limiting factor in the initial or continued use in most men is the fear of sticking a needle—no matter how small or painless—into the side of his penis.

HOW INTRACAVERNOUS INJECTIONS WORK

In the early 1980s, Virag first showed that the muscle relaxant drug papaverine, injected directly into the erectile tissue of the penis, could induce erection. Soon after Virag's discovery, other scientists found other families of drugs that could have similar effects, primarily certain alpha-blockers and prostaglandins.

This use of alpha-blocking drugs was discovered by Dr. Giles Brindley, a British neurologist and Olympic pole vaulter who played several musical instruments and spoke many languages. I happened to be in the first row at a lecture he gave in Las Vegas, Nevada, in 1983 to a packed audience of about 5,000 male and female physicians. It seemed strange that an elegant British doctor would be giving a formal lecture in a jogging suit. Dr. Brindley described the use of an alpha-blocking drug (drugs usually used to treat high blood pressure or benign prostate disease) and noted that when those drugs were injected into the penis, they caused long-lasting, rigid erections. To prove this assertion, Dr. Brindley stepped from the lectern, pulled down the jogging pants and walked through the audience, proudly displaying the rigid erection he had obtained by injecting himself before the lecture! It was a one-of-a-kind presentation that certainly proved his point to those of us in the audience.

Alpha-blocking drugs cause erections by relaxing the muscles around small blood vessels in the penis (and the rest of the body) and keeping them open. Alpha-blockers block the norepinephrine, a hormone that tightens muscles in the artery walls. Blocking the norepinephrine improves blood flow and lowers blood pressure. They can also help improve urine flow in older men with prostate problems. Remember, to be erect, the penis' smooth muscles must relax. When the effect of the norepinephrine is blocked, the smooth muscle cells will relax and an erection will ensue.

The next erection-producing drug used in ICI was first discovered by a Japanese urologist, also in 1983 (a banner year for erections worldwide).

The drug is known as prostaglandin E1, and when injected into the penis, it, too, can cause a longstanding, rigid erection. Similarly to the alpha-blockers, prostaglandin helps the smooth muscle cells relax to cause an erection. In this case, the drug increases production of a chemical called cyclic adenine monophosphate (cAMP), which causes the smooth muscle to relax.

The discovery of prostaglandin led to the creation of several injectible drugs that at the time (the late 80s into the mid-90s) were the only nonsurgical, FDA-approved ED treatments that actually worked. One of these drug products, called trimix, was sold in urologists' offices and is still used today. Trimix combines three drugs that cause erection: papaverine, prostaglandin E1, and a short-acting alpha-blocker, phentolamine. Each drug works through its own mechanism, and together they ensure that those smooth muscles relax.

ADVANTAGES AND DISADVANTAGES OF INTRACAVERNOUS INJECTION TREATMENT

Unlike the PDE-5 inhibitors, the man does not have to be sexually stimulated for the erection to occur with ICI treatment. That enables the man to inject himself about 20 to 30 minutes before he expects to have sex with his partner. Depending on the dose of the trimix given, the erection can last beyond the orgasm until the effect of the drug wears off (the erection will last whether or not you orgasm). With the help of his doctor, he and his partner can choose the correct dose to achieve the duration of erection that he desires. This can vary from 10 minutes to 4 hours depending on the wishes of the couple.

The ICI therapy works because it is locally injected and has primarily only a local effect—unlike the PDE-5 inhibitors, which affect many areas of the body, sometimes causing side effects that prohibit further use. Because of the focused dose of ICI, there is very little fear of interaction with other medications. There is essentially no medical reason not to use ICI, even in men taking nitroglycerin or blood thinners. I have prescribed ICI in men who were waiting for a heart transplant, and the drugs were used with no problems.

Cost is another positive factor. The ICI is obtained from a urologist's office or with a prescription from a urologist filled at a compounding pharmacy. (Those are pharmacies that "compound" or mix drugs that are not produced by the major drug companies.) The vials usually hold about 7.5 mL, and the charge for a vial is about $150 (charges vary). Because the amount of ICI injected varies for each person (as little as 0.01 mL up to 1 mL), the cost for each episode of intercourse is the least of any of the on-demand therapies. For example, if only 0.1 mL of trimix is needed (a typical dosage), you can have sex 50 times for that $150, or about $3.00 per episode of intercourse. Compare this to Viagra or similar drugs, which are over $20 per erection, and perhaps the idea of injecting yourself becomes more tolerable.

Another advantage is that ICI can be used indefinitely. I have had patients who have used an injection three or four times per week for nearly 25 years without a problem. However, as men age they may have reduced penile blood flow, increased tone in the penile smooth muscles, more hypertension, and worsening of diabetes and blood lipids, so that the ICI may become less effective over time. If those factors are not significant in an individual, then the ICI can continue to be used with gradual dose adjustments as needed.

The main problem with intracavernous injections is the *injection* part. A common response is, "Needles are for doctors to use, not normal people." Believe it or not, the procedure is nearly painless because you use a very fine needle that causes nearly no discomfort. Some men try ICI and it works, but they decide that intercourse is not worth the process of getting the drugs, storing them properly (usually in the refrigerator), and injecting themselves. I find that usually only the most motivated people continue to use the ICI method, despite having good results for most men.

SIDE EFFECTS AND RISKS

The duration of the erection depends on the volume of the drug injected: the more drug injected, the greater the chance of prolonged erection. Theoretically, after one injection, the resulting erection could last for days. But although having an erection for more than a day sounds great to some folks, it is really not a good idea. After more than 4 hours, toxic products begin to accumulate in the erect penis and can cause a great deal of pain, even eventually causing permanent scar tissue to form.

To avoid these harsh consequences, physicians stick to some basic rules to make sure the desired results occur:

1. Use the smallest volume of drug that gives the desired hardness and duration of erection.
2. Never inject more than one time per day. If the first injection does not work, come back another day.
3. If the dose does not give the desired result, move to higher dose in small increments and only under doctor's orders.

If the rules are followed, then there will never be a problem with prolonged erection.

A drawback of the drug prostaglandin is that in high doses it can stimulate the body's pain receptors and can cause local, aching pain throughout the entire penis. The discomfort does no damage to the penis, but some men find it distracts them from enjoying sex.

As another side effect, some men develop scar tissue in the penis, particularly if they inject the same area each time. It is best to use a different region of the penis with each injection. In some men, over time, the medication stops working because of changes that occur with aging or with diseases such as diabetes, hypertension, and hardening of the arteries. If that happens, his dose can be adjusted to achieve the same results. If that change eventually fails, then the patient probably needs to move up to a penile prosthetic implant to achieve dependable erections. In general, however, intracavernous injections are one of the safest and most effective treatments for ED.

A PATIENT'S STORY: INTRACAVERNOUS INJECTIONS

Arthur W. was a 69-year-old man, happily married for 48 years and in excellent health when he was diagnosed with a T1 localized prostate cancer. He had a PSA of 4.6 and a Gleason's 7 cancer. Sex was an important part of the couple's married life, and he elected to have a robotic radical nerve-sparing prostatectomy. The surgery was accomplished without problem. Urinary continence was obtained 2 months after surgery. At 3 months after surgery, he began to try different PDE-5 inhibitor drugs, all without effect. The couple rejected use of the VEDs and Muse, both of which proved ineffective in his case.

About 18 months after surgery, the couple came to my office. Arthur's PSA was undetectable and urinary continence was complete, but he was distressed. He fully expected to resume intercourse after the nerve-sparing surgery, and despite the couple's continued sexuality, he wanted to have sex with vaginal penetration. He had not known about ICI and was prepared for a penile prosthesis implantation. I introduced the topic of ICI as an alternative to an implant and explained that use of ICI did not burn any bridges: If after a while they did not want to continue with the injections, then he could still have the implant. After one test injection, the couple decided to use the therapy. He had responded to 0.2 mL of the trimix (a fairly low dose). Five months later, Arthur returned for a second vial of the trimix. He was ecstatic with the results—not only had ICI allowed he and his wife to fully resume their sex life, but it had returned his sense of "maleness" that he had lost.

Muse, Another Drug Treatment for Erectile Dysfunction

In 1995, the FDA approved the medication Muse to treat ED. It was highly successful its first year (with $120 million in sales), until Viagra was introduced the following year. Muse is also a prostaglandin-based product but is not swallowed or injected. Instead, the patient places a rice grain-sized prostaglandin medication into the opening of his urethra, about ½ to 1 inch up the penis, about 20 minutes before intercourse. The drug is absorbed into the veins around the urethra, some of which drain into the erectile bodies.

The prostaglandin then creates an erection through the same mechanism as it does when injected and, like ICI, can work even there is some post-operative nerve damage. The difference is the amount of prostaglandin needed: Muse comes in doses of 250, 500, or 1000 μg. With an injection, the maximum dose is 40 μg. The reason so much more drug is needed is because only a fraction of the drug gets into the penile erectile tissue. To make the drug more effective, a specially designed rubber band is placed around the base of the penis.

Of the men who use the two highest doses of Muse (500 and 1000 μg), 30% to 50% get an erection hard enough for vaginal penetration. The side effects, including penile pain and burning in 31% of patients and a drop in blood pressure in another 6%, limit its overall use to about 20% of the men who try it.[2,3]

Vacuum Devices

Vacuum erection devices (VEDs) were developed in the 1980s, before the introduction of the PDE-5 inhibitors or ICI, but after the successful unveiling of penile implants (next section of this chapter). VEDs offer a non-surgical, effective alternative for men with ED after prostate therapy. Unlike other non-surgical treatments, it is a mechanical, rather than pharmaceutical, fix.

How Vacuum Devices Work

The VEDs consist of two parts: a plastic cylindrical sheath attached to a small motor or lever and a "rubber band"-like tourniquet. The plastic sheath is placed over the penis to create a negative pressure (literally a vacuum) around the penis, pulling blood into the erectile bodies. (*See* Figure 4.2.) The vacuum is created with a motor (in more expensive models) or by cranking a lever (in more basic models). After the penis becomes rigid with blood, a tourniquet is placed around the base of the penis to hold the extra blood in place, and the plastic tube used to create the vacuum is pulled away. Intercourse can then take place with a 30-minute time limit because of the tourniquet (wouldn't want to leave that on too long!) The vacuum can only be created if there is a tight seal between the lower abdomen and the base of the plastic cylinder. That is accomplished by applying a lubricant gel to the abdomen and the tube. Shaving or trimming the pubic hair can also help increase the vacuum seal.

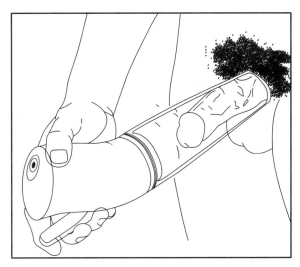

Figure 4.2 This is how a vacuum erection device is used. The clear plastic cylinder is placed over the flaccid penis. A jelly to create a good air seal is placed on the end of the tube that rests on the lower abdomen. With the aid of a motorized or hand-manipulated vacuum pump, a vacuum is created in the tube around the penis, drawing blood into the penis. When an erection is obtained, a tourniquet is placed around the base of the penis. The vacuum is released and the tube removed, leaving the erect penis. The tourniquet can be left in place for 30 minutes without injury to the penis.
(Reprinted with permission from *Timm Medical Technoloiges, Inc.*)

SIDE EFFECTS AND RISKS

The VED is a very safe device with few risks. Some people have pain when the vacuum is created and the blood is drawn into the penile chambers. The head of the penis may appear blue and swollen after a while, because of the tourniquet, which may also cause the penis to feel a little cold or numb. Other men may have some bruising or reddish pinpoint-size dots on their skin. Although unpleasant, these side effects are harmless and disappear after a day or two at the most.

It is important to use devices that are manufactured by FDA-approved companies. To obtain reimbursement from your insurance company, you need a doctor's prescription. However, they can be purchased online without one, should your insurance not cover the expense. A recent review of one Internet site showed four brands for sale—Erecaid, Encore, Vitality, and Eros, ranging in price from $95 to $375. The companies that charge more, such as the brands named above, offer more supportive service and guidance should there be a problem with the device. The less expensive VEDs sold for a low price in "adult" stores or on the Internet do not have an important safety feature: a maximal

A PATIENT'S STORY: VACUUM DEVICES

David B. is a 73-year-old man who had been treated for localized prostate cancer 2 years ago. He had erections for the first year after therapy, but then he became unable to achieve sufficient erection to consummate sex. His family doctor had prescribed Viagra but he did not want to use the drug because he was concerned about side effects and his particular insurance did not cover the high cost. His wife was 76 years old; they were married for 50 years and had a long and happy sexual relationship. They had continued to be sexual with one another after his ED began but wanted to have occasional coitus as well. I offered them ICI, but he was afraid to inject himself, so they settled on a try with the VED. I wrote a prescription, and they obtained the device from a surgical supply house that ordered it from the manufacturer. David had some problems with using the VED at first (he didn't apply enough lubricant to create the vacuum seal) but I taught him the correct method during an office visit, and after that, things went smoothly. He and his wife have intercourse once a month with the aid of the VED and are satisfied.

negative pressure valve that is found in the better VEDs. If the valve is missing, then very high pressures can be obtained, damaging blood vessels and causing bruising and pain in the penis. It is best to use the approved devices.

The principal problems with the VEDs are the mechanical nature of creating erection, the sloppiness of the gels needed to obtain a sufficient seal, the discomfort of the tourniquet, and the lack of complete penile rigidity in most patients. In my experience, these devices have the best success in older couples with a longstanding relationship for whom sex is an occasional event and in whom the other options are either deemed impractical or unsafe. The lack of a truly rigid erection (but usually "erect enough") coupled with the safety of the device is an acceptable compromise to those who use them.

PERMANENT, SURGICAL SOLUTIONS TO ERECTILE DYSFUNCTION: PENILE IMPLANTS

In the early days of ED treatment, researchers were inspired to replicate a feature of certain non-human mammals like bears, cats, and hedgehogs, all of whom have a bone in the penis. Early in the twentieth century, surgeons tried to correct ED in humans by placing rib bone or cartilage into the erectile bodies.

The experiment failed because over time the cartilage was re-absorbed by the body. In the 1940s, Willard Goodwin, a doctor at the Johns Hopkins Medical Center, had a dentist friend who worked with a new plastic, methacrylate, that was neither re-absorbed nor rejected by the body. Goodwin used this new plastic to develop a prosthesis for his patients who had been treated with urethral cancer. The problem was that methacrylate is rigid and does not bend, so the device was uncomfortable to have in place or to use for intercourse. It was used in a few men but never really caught on. Today, advanced technology and materials have made prostheses more comfortable and are used in thousands of men with ED of various causes.

There are two types of penile implants: semi-rigid and inflatable.

Semi-Rigid Implant

The big breakthrough in penile implants came with the invention of medical-grade silicone. Silicone is not rejected by the body and, unlike methacrylate, is bendable. Robert Pearman, a urologist in Encino, California, invented a penile implant in the mid-1960s using flexible silicone. It was a single flat rod that fit into the visible portion of the penis and afforded enough rigidity to allow vaginal penetration. For the first time, urologists could offer a successful therapy to men with ED that was durable and safe. If the man was willing to have surgery, then he and his partner could reclaim their sex life. As with modern penile prostheses, the device allowed successful spontaneous sex without planning in advance, as is required with all other therapies.

The device worked well for several years in many people but was supplanted in the early 70s by a more anatomically accurate invention from two industrious urologists from South Florida, Drs. Hernion Carrion and Michael Small. The Small–Carrion prosthesis used a more durable form of silicone and not one, but two rods to completely fill the erectile bodies on both sides (*see* Fig. 4.3 for a modern version of the Small-Carrion prosthesis). The implant allowed satisfactory intercourse, was bendable, and was more comfortable for the man and his partner.

The semi-rigid implants require no effort from the patient other than bending them into the desired position for intercourse. For that reason, they are also called *malleable prostheses* because the interior of the devices are composed of materials that when bent assume the position into which they are bent. I have also heard them referred to as "gooseneck lamp"-style implants. They can be bent up to have intercourse or bent down to be contained in one's pants without being seen. They always remain with the same length, diameter, and hardness. Despite the constant erection, which seems a drawback to men before surgery, the bendability of the device prevents the embarrassment of a rigid erection poking out of

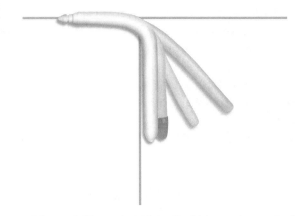

Figure 4.3 Four of the available semi-rigid (malleable) prostheses. Each can be bent into a flexed position so that clothing can be worn. To have intercourse, the prosthesis is lifted into a straight line to affect vaginal penetration. There are no moving parts or extraneous tubes. The penis is always the same length and diameter, only the position of the penis is changed.
(Reprinted with permission. Courtesy of American Medical Systems®, Inc.)

A Patient's Story: Semi-Rigid Penile Implant

Juan J. was an unmarried 57-year-old man who had a radical retropubic nerve-sparing prostatectomy. He took medication for his mild diabetes and hypertension. He was sexually active with several girlfriends prior to his prostatectomy, but 2 years after his surgery, he was unable to achieve erection sufficient for intercourse with any of the PDE-5 inhibitor drugs. He was terrified of using ICI therapy and flatly refused. The next option offered was a penile prosthesis. Juan was quite certain that he did not want to inflate the prosthesis and chose a semi-rigid device. He had mild problems with tightness of the foreskin and had a simultaneous circumcision. The prosthesis was placed through that incision so there was no extra scar to explain to his female companions. Post-operatively, he had more pain than he expected for the first several weeks after surgery. He also complained that the erect penis before surgery had been larger than it was with the prosthesis. Men should be told in advance that radical prostatectomy may cause a slight decrease in size of the penis (see page 123) and that they should be prepared for that event before the prosthesis is placed. After 6 months, Juan was having satisfactory intercourse but still complained about mild pain at the tip of his penis. By 1 year after surgery, that pain disappeared and he stated that he had a good sex life with the implant.

one's pants when dressed. They are fully concealable—men who have them simply bend the penis flat against their bodies to conceal the stiffness.

Inflatable Implant

Also in the mid-70s, the first successful inflatable penile implant was developed, followed a decade later by a second, more rigid model.

The inflatable implant is contained entirely within the body and not visible to onlookers. The inflatable penile implant uses the shifting of salt water from a reservoir in the scrotum into cylinders placed in the penis' cavernous bodies. The liquid is shifted by the man himself, when he feels ready to have sex, by a hand-powered squeeze pump in the scrotum (*see* Figure 4.4). The use of liquid

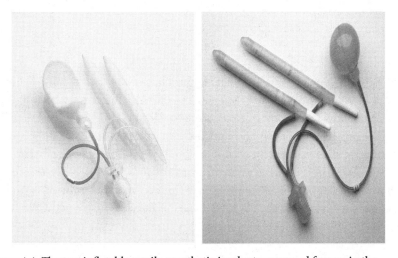

Figure 4.4 The two inflatable penile prosthetic implants approved for use in the United States. On the left is the Coloplast Titan® OTR device, and on the right side is the American Medical Systems 700® with an inhibizone antibiotic coating (the dark color). Each product is constructed with a material that is not rejected by the body (polyurethane) for the Coloplast Titan® OTR and Silicone for the AMS 700®.
For each device, the two cylinders are placed in the corporal bodies, the pump goes in the scrotum, and the reservoir is placed in the space in front of the bladder in the abdomen. The devices contain salt water that is shifted between the reservoir and the cylinders. The energy for moving the fluid between sites is provided by the user, who must squeeze the pump.
(Reprinted with permission. Courtesy of American Medical Systems®, Inc. and Coloplast, Inc.).

makes the implant a hydraulic system, and therefore the inflated penis is neither bendable nor compressible. That translates into a very rigid penis when fully erect. When ready for intercourse, the man squeezes the small pump, forcing fluid into the cylinders. Each full squeeze forces about a teaspoonful of salt water into the cylinders. The number of squeezes needed depends on the size of the penis. The larger your penis, the more pumping you need to do. When the pressure in the penis cylinders is at its max, no further fluid will enter, so you don't have to worry about overpumping or bursting the cylinders (or the penis—a fear many men seem to have).

After the sexual act is complete, the newest inflatable devices have a button on the pump (concealed under the skin) to press to empty the fluid out of the cylinders and back into the reservoir. Although the cylinders become soft when the fluid empties, their length stays the same. So the flaccid (non-erect) penis length is always the same as the erect "final product"—this is also true for the semi-rigid penile implants. For a man who has a big difference (pre-implant) between his flaccid and erect penis length, there is good news: his penis will always be its longer, erect length after his implant.

Risks and Side Effects

For both the semi-rigid and inflatable prostheses, the prime complication is infection. The prostheses are not capable of resisting the bacteria found on the skin (staphylococcus), and effort is taken by all implanting surgeons to minimize the possibility of such an infection. The infection rate for either implant is about 3% in non-diabetic men and about 8% in men with diabetes. If an infection occurs, usually the entire implant has to be removed. If the infection is of a particular type of *Staph*, then the surgeon may recommend a "salvage procedure" a removal of the device with an antibiotic washout of the prosthesis bed, followed by replacement of the device.

Also, over time (usually a decade or more), the inflatable implants can experience mechanical failure in about 10% of cases. If this happens, then the implant can be removed and replaced for another decade or so of erections.

Factors in Deciding Which Implant to Use

In the United States, most insurance covers the cost of penile prosthetic implantation, so that the choice of which implant to have placed does not depend on cost for the consumer. (The inflatable prosthesis is about twice the cost of a semi-rigid device—$9,000 vs. $5,500—if not paid for by insurance.)

Patients often ask me which implant style I think would be best for them. I respond by asking them their favorite color. There is, of course, no "best"

A PATIENT'S STORY: INFLATABLE PENILE IMPLANT

Paul C. was a 39-year-old man who had experienced lifelong ED, when his girl-friend persuaded him to attend an Impotence Anonymous meeting at a local hospital. One of the other men there recommended that Paul see me. At his appointment, I did a few tests and then explained the implant options. "The one that pumped up seemed like the way to go," said Paul. "It seemed more realistic, maybe. I think it was more expensive, so I thought it might be better!"

He remembers being in quite a bit of pain after the surgery; he took a week off from work to recover afterward—and recommends prune juice during the 6 weeks of recovery to avoid any straining during the healing time. "I remember waking up afterward and seeing the erection, thinking, 'Wow! This is really worth it!'"

Paul's first prosthetic lasted 15 years, and he just had a second surgery last year to put in his second implant. He has found that time has helped him become very comfortable with his implant and he is now "totally open and unembarrassed" about it. He says he finds it is indistinguishable from a normal erection: before sex he just goes to the bathroom and pumps it up; afterward, he presses the flat, square button under his skin and the erection goes down. "There's no reason you actually have to say anything at first—depending on the relationship—as it's not obvious at all. No woman I've been with has ever been repelled. Every one I've spoken to about it has listened attentively and said 'OK, fine.' It's really not an issue."

After years of half-hearted attempts to get help for his ED (he even visited a sex therapist and tried a sexual surrogate—a sex therapist who has sex with her clients to help them achieve therapeutic goals)—Paul found not just a good therapy, but an (almost) permanent cure with the inflatable implant. "It's been a real life-changer for me," says Paul. "The only thing I would have done differently is I wish I had started the process much earlier."

color for everyone, as there is no "best" prosthesis for every patient. In my experience of 40 years of placing penile prostheses, I have learned that some men simply do not like the concept of "pumping" themselves up. They are terrified of having to squeeze their scrotum to inflate themselves to full penile rigidity. Those men and others who have decreased strength in their dominant hand, who are very clumsy with their hands, or who are obese and would have trouble reaching the scrotum should be advised to choose a semi-rigid device.

The surgery takes slightly longer for the inflatable device, because of the placement of the pump. However, the inflatable gives superior rigidity in most cases, but for men with a wide diameter penis, the semi-rigid prosthesis gives good enough rigidity for satisfactory vaginal penetration. Men who shower in a public locker room might not want to have a semi-rigid device with its full erection in plain view of other gym members.

Urinary Incontinence after Prostate Cancer

Urinary incontinence (UI) is the second most common complication of prostate cancer treatment, and can be every bit as devastating to the patient's quality of life as erectile dysfunction (ED). Urinary incontinence is the inability to control one's urine flow. For some men, this means that they may have some leaking of urine when they experience increased pressure on the bladder (as with coughing, sneezing, or sitting down or standing up); this is known as *stress urinary incontinence* (SUI). In other cases, the need to urinate may arise so suddenly and severely that the bladder empties on its own; this is known as *urge urinary incontinence* (UUI). If either stress or urge incontinence gets so bad that urine leaks more or less continuously, then it is known as total incontinence.

Almost every patient has some incontinence immediately after prostate surgery. This is because the prostate provides some support for blocking the flow of urine and when it is removed, the urinary sphincter muscle has to do the job by itself. It usually takes about 3 months after surgery before most patients return to continence (it can take up to 24 months). If you are experiencing incontinence after surgery, make sure you talk about it with your surgeon during follow-up appointments, as there may be temporary treatments to ease your problems while you heal. If incontinence problems do not ease up after 6 months to a year, it is likely you require additional treatment to recover.

Incontinence can come as a bewildering shock because most of us don't think twice about urinating—it seems to happen automatically and require little or no thought. In reality, the act of voiding (urinating or peeing)—particularly in men—is a highly complex physical act, requiring the cooperation of the brain, spinal cord, nerves, the bladder, the prostate and the urethra, and the muscle tissue known as the urinary sphincter.

ANOTHER ANATOMY LESSON

The urinary system allows the body to dispose of liquid waste or urine. (Solid waste products move through the intestines and out the anus as stool.) The kidneys, twin organs at the small of your back, filter out waste material from your blood and send urine down to the bladder through tubes known as ureters. The bladder stores the urine until it is time to urinate, then urine exits out the bladder neck, through the prostate and out the penis via another tube called the urethra.

The bladder is a hollow organ in your pelvis that stretches from an empty balloon to a grapefruit-sized sac when full. Like the penis, the bladder is made up mostly of smooth muscle tissue—muscles that cannot be controlled by thinking about them. There is one muscle in the bladder that you can control, however. The urinary, or urethral, sphincter is a circular muscle, like a rubber band, that tightens around the urethra to stop the flow of urine. You can consciously tighten this muscle when you are in the middle of urinating and stop your flow. The bladder neck is the portion of the bladder attached to the prostate; the bladder neck is closed unless you are urinating. Cutting through the prostate is a section of the urethra called the prostatic urethra. Urine passes through this section of urethra on its way out of the body; the prostatic urethra is also where semen enters the urethra during sex. Right where the urethra exits the prostate is the portion of the urethra surrounded by the urinary sphincter and closed by the sphincter muscle, unless we are in the act of urinating. The urethra continues past the sphincter and out the tip of the penis, where urine and semen leave the body. (*See* Figure 5.1 for a partial diagram of the male urinary system.)

When the bladder becomes full (about 15 ounces of urine), the brain is made aware through nerve signals from the bladder. In an infant, the brains responds with a signal to the bladder to make it contract, and the baby urinates into his or her diaper. Through the process of toilet training, a child learns to void at specific times into the toilet. This conscious urination is a process of the nerve signal being received by the brain and the person making a decision to urinate or not, depending on whether or not they are in a bathroom. When an adult

Side view

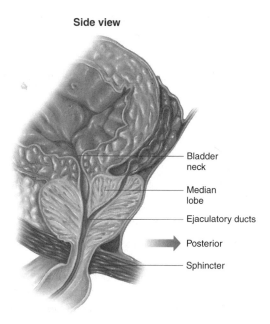

- Bladder neck
- Median lobe
- Ejaculatory ducts
- Posterior
- Sphincter

Figure 5.1 The relationship of the prostate, urethra, and external sphincter muscle to the bladder and bladder neck from the side. The sketch is a representation of a man with a mildly enlarged prostate and a thickened bladder.
(Courtesy of American Medical Systems ®, Minnetonka, Minnesota; www.americanmedicalsystems.com.)

decides to urinate, he contracts his bladder and at the same time the smooth muscles of the bladder neck and prostate relax, allowing urine to flow out of the bladder via the urethra.

The urinary sphincter is about one-third the thickness of your little finger. It is composed of both *skeletal muscle cells* and *non-voluntary smooth muscle cells*. You can control skeletal muscles, like the muscle cells in your biceps that allow you to flex your arm when you want. Non-voluntary smooth muscle cells are those, like the muscles in the penis, which you cannot consciously control. It is the sphincter muscle that allows you to stop your urinary stream while you are urinating. When a man urinates, not only does his bladder contract but the smooth muscle cells of the bladder neck, prostate, and the urinary sphincter all must relax also. When the bladder is empty, the reverse happens: The sphincter contracts, the prostate and the bladder neck contract, and the bladder itself relaxes in preparation for its refilling with urine over time. All of those actions are mediated through properly functioning muscles and nerve fibers. Even a small disruption of nerves and/or muscle cells can cause an imbalance in proper urinary control.

CAUSES OF URINARY INCONTINENCE AFTER PROSTATE CANCER TREATMENT

Urinary incontinence and other bladder complications can arise after prostate cancer treatment for a number of reasons, including:

1. problems that exist prior to treatment, which are only discovered after the prostate is removed
2. your age at the time of treatment (about 10% greater chance of UI in patients older than age 70 years, when compared to patients younger than age 50)
3. extension of the cancer into the urinary sphincter
4. experience and expertise of the surgeon or radiotherapist
5. bad luck.

Urinary incontinence of several degrees (irritation to total loss of control) is a known complication for all kinds of prostate cancer treatment. Fortunately, most men do not have a lasting problem with UI after treatment for prostate cancer. In a landmark quality-of-life study, 80% of prostate cancer survivors reported no incontinence issues (the number is slightly worse if non-nerve-sparing surgery was done). Similarly, 90% of men reported no incontinence after either type of radiation. Ninety-five percent of men had no issues with urinary irritation (urgency and/or frequency) after surgery, and about 80% had no issues after either brachytherapy or radiotherapy. [1]

After Surgery

The prostate sits directly between the bladder and the urinary sphincter muscles. Because of this position, the prostate helps control urinary continence. During a prostatectomy for prostate cancer, the prostate gland is removed (as shown in Fig. 5.2 A & B). The space in which the prostate existed cannot be left open or urine would not be able to pass out of the body (as shown in Fig. 5.2B).

The surgeon carefully re-attaches the bladder to the urethra and the urinary sphincter, as shown in Figure 5.2C. After a radical prostatectomy, the urinary sphincter now lies just outside the bladder neck.

Pre-surgery, the sphincter muscle compresses the urethra (through which men urinate) and blocks the entire urethral opening, keeping the urine in the bladder until there is an urge to void and relaxation of the sphincter muscle occurs. After surgery, this muscle is too weak in some men to compress the urethra at first (it has been "lazy" since the prostate gland was doing some of

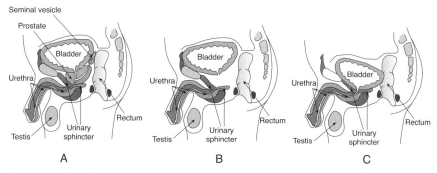

Figure 5.2 The relationship of the normal anatomy of the prostate bladder and urethra before (A), during (B), and after (C), a radical prostatectomy. In (B), the bladder and seminal vesicles have been removed, and in (C) the bladder is anastomosed to the urethra adjacent to the external sphincter. (Courtesy of Kelvin Davies, Ph.D.)

this job). Men can "wake up" and strengthen their urinary sphincters before and after surgery (as soon as the catheter has been removed) with Kegel-type exercises (*see* page 98). Usually after a few months of these exercises, the sphincter becomes stronger and more effectively seals the opening to prevent urine leakage. Unfortunately, in some cases, it is not that easy, and urinary continence does not return fully or at all.

PRE-EXISTING PROBLEMS CAN BE DISCOVERED AFTER SURGERY

As discussed earlier, the continence mechanism is a combination of the strength of the bladder contraction resisted by the strength of the urinary sphincter. Before treatment, the presence of an enlarged prostate may have restricted the outflow of urine easily and kept the man in total urinary control even in the presence of a weakened urinary sphincter. Such a weakened sphincter muscle in that state is less effective in controlling urine when the prostate is removed. Also, the enlarged prostate can hide incontinence problems by blocking the urine leaks. After the prostate is removed, the existing urinary incontinence no longer faces a "road block," and the leaking begins.

Another cause of UI after prostatectomy could be damage to the urethra, urinary sphincter, or nearby nerves during the surgery. These areas could be nicked or disturbed, diminishing their strength or effectiveness. The nerves are especially hard to see during surgery; therefore, I recommend any surgical approach that improves the surgeon's field of vision (such as robotic).

After Radiation

Once again, as with ED, UI arrives at different times with the different therapies. When radiation therapy is given, whether using seeds or external beam (EBRT), incontinence can begin after about a month and can worsen over time. In general, incontinence is rarer after radiation than after surgery but can still occur—most often in the form of urge incontinence.

Incontinence after radiation treatment is a result of radiation damage to the organs, nerves, or muscles involved with urination. As discussed in Chapter 2, radiation cannot be precisely pinpointed to only cancer cells, and there is bound to be at least a little bit of collateral damage during treatment. Radiation damage to the urinary sphincter muscle will cause stress incontinence (SUI); damage to the bladder or bladder neck may bring on urge incontinence (UUI). In either of these cases, if the damage is severe enough (perhaps if the man had extensive cancer and therefore higher doses of radiation) then the radiation can also cause total incontinence.

As in surgery, radiation can cause direct damage to the urinary sphincter. Radiation seeds might be placed close enough to the sphincter muscle to injure the muscle cells, or external beam therapy might be aimed to hit a tumor that is especially close to the urinary sphincter. In either case, the sphincter can be scarred or otherwise damaged, so that it does not close properly. Inadvertent injury of the nerve fibers that run alongside the prostate to the sphincter muscle can also occur with radiation, further limiting the effectiveness of urine control. Figure 5.3 contrasts a healthy urinary sphincter with one which has been damaged, causing UI.

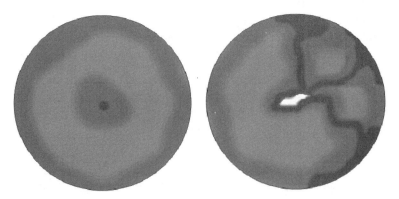

Figure 5.3 The image on the left shows the normal appearance of the urethral sphincter when looking at it through the lens of a cystscope placed in the penis. The image on the right shows a sphincter that has been damaged and is scarred in an open position so that urine can continually leak out. (Courtesy of Kelvin Davies, Ph.D.)

Total Urinary Incontinence

Total urinary incontinence is one of the most potentially demoralizing problems a man may face after prostate cancer treatment. It occurs most often after surgery but can occur rarely after either EBRT or brachytherapy if there is a complication of the radiation. If it occurs after surgery, then total urinary incontinence does so immediately but usually improves with time; with radiation, the reverse is true, and a case of incontinence may continue to worsen over the months after treatment.

The probability of total urinary incontinence varies, depending on the kind of treatment given, the amount of cancer present before treatment, and whether or not more than one therapy is given to treat the disease. For example, the rate of incontinence will be different if your cancer is a low-grade tumor that is localized to the prostate, as opposed to a more aggressive, high-grade tumor that may extend into other tissues such as the bladder neck.

Surgery is responsible for the majority of cases of total urinary incontinence, because of direct injury to the sphincter muscle or the nerves that control it. As noted above, the prostate gland offers resistance to the flow of urine. Because the connection between the prostate and urethra is removed during radical prostatectomy, the external sphincter becomes the primary urinary control mechanism, and if it is damaged or weakened, then the urine can continuously drip from the bladder and come out the penis. If this happens, then the patient may need to wear continence pads for comfort and hygiene and might consider some of the UI treatments listed in the Chapter 6 to provide a more permanent fix.

Total incontinence can occur after extensive radiation, too, but through a slightly different process. In those cases, the prostate is intact but usually scarred

Table 5.1. TYPES OF URINARY INCONTINENCE

Type of incontinence	Definition	Cause
Total	Always dripping: a degree of urge or stress incontinence	Severe damage to or weakening of the urethral sphincter muscle caused by surgery or (rarely) radiation.
Urge	Need to know where the bathroom is located at all times; leaking caused by sudden, urgent need to urinate.	Bladder injury or a change in bladder muscles or nerves, usually caused by radiation.
Stress	Dripping caused by coughing, sneezing, or changing position.	Age; damage to or weakening of the urinary sphincter muscle caused by surgery or radiation.

and less flexible because of the treatment. If the external sphincter is similarly damaged by the treatment, then the patient can experience an inability to control the urine as after radical prostatectomy, because the sphincter will no longer form a tight seal around the urethra. The result can be a continuous dripping of urine. Each of these conditions can be effectively treated with surgical methods so that urinary control will be regained.

Stress Incontinence

For 88% of the men who have UI post-treatment, they suffer from stress incontinence, which means they experience urinary leakage with the increased abdominal pressure associated with coughing, sneezing, laughing, and sitting and standing. In these patients, the sphincter forms a seal around the urethra but not a tight enough one to keep urine from dripping when the pressure is raised in the bladder.

When a person coughs, sneezes, or even laughs heartily, the pressure in the abdomen is greatly increased. The pressure wave is transferred first to the bladder wall, then to the interior of the bladder. If that pressure is higher than the pressure of the sphincter's seal around the urethra, then the person will leak a spurt of urine. That can happen with any action that increases abdominal pressure, such as sit-ups or heavy lifting. If the problem is minor, with only a few drops of urine leaking out, then most men simply use some type of urinary pad in their underwear. For many men, this is a temporary measure until they do enough pelvic floor exercises to strengthen their sphincter muscles. Some men use pads as a "just-in-case" method of protection, even though they do not need them every day.

Stress incontinence is the most common type of incontinence to develop after radical prostatectomy. It is experienced after surgery by nearly all patients for at least a few weeks. In some, it endures longer and requires additional treatment to cure. The patient quality-of-life study referenced above showed that by 2 years after surgery, 20% of men used pads, 5% used pads after EBRT, and 8% after brachytherapy.[2]

Urge Urinary Incontinence

Like SUI, urge urinary incontinence (UUI) is not constant. As its name suggests, urge incontinence usually includes a frequent and urgent need to urinate. It can also mean occasional leakage resulting from spasms in the bladder or urinary sphincter muscles.

When UUI happens, the smooth muscle cells of the bladder contract when they are not supposed to and that causes a sudden squirt of urine. It is not known why that contraction occurs, and therefore, the treatments for the problem are non-specific to the bladder cells and as a result are fraught with poor results and significant side effects.

In men with urge urinary incontinence, the uncontrollable need to urinate is the primary problem. Urge urinary incontinence occurs in about 12% of the men who have urinary incontinence after radical prostatectomy. Perhaps there was an element of urgency present before the radical prostatectomy, but a normal urinary sphincter was able to prevent the undesired flow of urine and the man could stay dry. After surgery, when the prostate is no longer present to partially block the flow of urine, an added burden is placed on the urinary sphincter. When the involuntary contractions are stronger than the strength of the sphincter to resist the increased bladder pressure, then urine leakage occurs.

Bladder Neck Contracture

Another cause of UUI is a blockage of urine flow that sometimes happens during post-operative healing. The blockage is referred to as a bladder neck contracture. When the bladder is joined to the urethra after the prostate is removed, the two organs must heal together. In a small percentage of men, the bladder neck contracts a little too much during healing, and the ensuing blockage causes the bladder to be overactive. The opening of the bladder can be as small as a pinhole. The diagnosis of bladder neck contracture should be suspected if the man has to push hard to urinate after the surgery or if the urinary stream is very slow. Sometimes the opening is so small that the man cannot urinate at all. That is called urinary retention and must be treated by stretching the opening. In other cases, the patient doesn't recognize his stream is slowed; luckily, most urologists can easily measure the rate of urine flow. The normal urine flow is about 16 mL per second. Men with bladder neck contractions may be voiding at a rate of only 3 or 4 mL per second. The bladder works so hard to empty itself that the muscles of the bladder wall become thickened and irritated and the entire bladder begins to show signs of bladder overactivity: urinary urgency, frequency, and incontinence.

Urethral Stricture

Similarly to bladder neck contracture, a urethral stricture can develop after treatment and obstruct the urine flow. During the prostatectomy, surgical instruments may graze the urethra, or the urinary catheter that is left in place after the surgery may irritate this delicate tube. The resulting irritation of the urethra can cause a narrowing of the urethral tube in the form of a urethral stricture.

No matter whether the stricture is in the bladder neck or the urethra, the bladder's response is to push harder against the obstruction, which can wear on the bladder muscles and an overactive bladder may result—with eventual urgency and in severe cases UUI. As for bladder neck contracture, the treatment for a urethral stricture is also surgical: using radial cuts of the inner circle of the urethra in several places while looking at the urethra through a cystoscope. If there is no recurrence within 6 months after treatment, most are considered cured.

A PATIENT'S STORY: URINARY INCONTINENCE AFTER SURGERY

Richard D. was 52 years old when he was diagnosed with prostate cancer. "My first 52 years I was invincible; cancer was something that happened to someone else." His prostatectomy was successful in that the cancer was gone, but Richard was troubled by bad incontinence afterward. Luckily because of his business he could wear scrubs, and the baggy pant legs hid the collection bag of his catheter. The 3 months it took to recover from the surgery were exhausting for him. He couldn't drive or lift anything; his children wanted to help; and his wife drove him everywhere. Richard remembers this time as "a totally emasculating process."

Richard is one of the unlucky men whose incontinence was not resolved with further treatment. Because of a surgeon's mistake, an attempt to correct his incontinence with an artificial urinary sphincter ended up making matters worse. Today he wears incontinence pads and he endures as best he can.

"Every couple of months I will tell my wife: 'I am so damn tired of this.' But it's the fate I have and it's a lot better than the alternative [dying of cancer]. This friend and I kid each other that the only pants we have are black or navy because you never know when you're going to leak. It seems like your bladder gets smaller—when you stand up, you often leak . . . trying to be nonchalant, walking to the bathroom. . . You say a couple expletives and go back to your dinner and hope your pants dry before you get to the theater. It's frustrating. It's embarrassing. But there's really nothing else."

OTHER URINARY COMPLICATIONS OF PROSTATE CANCER TREATMENT

Although stress incontinence is by far the most prevalent of urinary complications post-prostate cancer treatment, there are other side effects from surgery or radiation that can affect the proper functioning of the urinary system.

Overactive Bladder

Urinary incontinence may occur along with overactive bladder (OAB), a syndrome that is a combination of a sudden and urgent need to urinate, urinary frequency, urination at night (nocturia), and urinary urge incontince. OAB can be caused by problems with the bladder muscles, bladder disease, or prostate disease (such as an enlarged prostate or prostate cancer). OAB is present in about 43 million men and women in the United States, about 16% of the population. In men, OAB is usually associated with benign prostatic enlargement (32% of male OAB patients) or bladder neck contracture (22%). In one study, it was found that 20% of men with OAB had had a radical prostatectomy earlier.[3] After a radical prostatectomy, there is usually some weakening of the urinary sphincter, and a man who's never had any symptoms of OAB may now have incontinence because his prostate is no longer in place to help control urine flow.

Overactive bladder may also occur after radiation therapy for prostate cancer. Radiation can irritate the bladder tissues and therefore increase the number of incontinence episodes, even in the presence of an intact urinary sphincter. That happens because the force of the contraction of the bladder wall is so high that the sphincter, although appropriately closed, cannot contain the urine.

If you are still having urinary urgency several months after cancer treatment that doesn't seem to respond to Kegel exercises and is not SUI, then you might have OAB.

TREATMENT FOR OVERACTIVE BLADDER

The treatment of OAB caused by bladder neck contracture is surgery to correct the contracture. This surgery can be done through the penis so that another incision does not have to be made (fortunately the procedure is done under general anesthesia). The instrument called a "resectoscope" has a bright light and good lens system that allows the urologist to see the actual obstruction on a video screen. The obstruction is corrected by making tiny cuts in the contracture in several places with a laser. The cuts allow the inner circumference of the bladder neck to open up, increasing the radius of the opening leading to the urethra and restoring normal urine flow. Milder OAB can be treated with medication; more on that in the Chapter 6.

Bladder Irritation

Both radiation seeds and external beam radiation can cause changes in the bladder wall that irritate the bladder and make it more sensitive, so that it contracts more often than normal. This can cause urinary urgency and, in severe cases, UUI. After brachytherapy, 18% of men experience bladder irritation; after EBRT, about 14% of patients have this problem.[4] Unlike post-prostatectomy problems, this side effect can worsen with time, as radiation has a cumulative and increasing effect over the first year after the treatment. The peak of such problems occurs at 2 years post-treatment.

RISK OF URINARY INCONTINENCE AFTER TREATMENT

As noted above, UI is a known complication of any prostate cancer treatment. The reported range of UI in the medical literature varies quite widely depending on who is doing the reporting. Even definitions of incontinence vary from report to report, making it difficult to compare one report with another. Each of those factors must be accounted for when trying to make a therapy decision that relies on statistical data.

One study that evaluated men who had a prostatectomy for localized disease found that before surgery, 3.6% of the men reported frequent urinary leakage or no control.[5] The numbers were highest 6 months after surgery, when 25% of men gave that report. The percent of incontinent post-operative patients decreased to about 10.4% at 2 years. Interestingly, the numbers increased slightly to 13.9% at 5 years after surgery. That increase may happen because men forget that they need to continue to do pelvic floor exercises throughout life, because as soon as the sphincter muscle weakens, the incontinence or leaking can return.

In another study of 3,477 men who had an open radical prostatectomy done by a highly experienced surgeon, the incontinence rate was 7%.[6] (It should be noted that this rate of incontinence, because of the excellence of the surgeon, should represent the lowest rate of expected UI. Other surgeons with less experience may have a higher rate of post-operative UI.) As it does in return of erectile function, age makes a difference in bladder control. The continence rate was 95% in men younger than age 50 years and 86% in men age 70 years or older. Most men in the study were between 60 and 69 years of age, with a continence rate of 93% for that age group. When controlled for nerve-sparing surgery, Gleason's score, pre-operative PSA, or post-operative radiation, age was the most significant variable. Other studies have shown that men who require removal of both erectile nerves because they have more extensive cancer have a higher rate of incontinence.

Although the reported incidence of any UI after prostatectomy is reported over the wide range of to 2% to 87%, it is my experience that about 10% of surgery patients are incontinent (i.e., need to wear pads) when the surgery is done by an experienced surgeon. The reported incidence of UI is 16% after radiation seeds and 11% after EBRT. In other words, all of the treatments for prostate cancer offer about the same chance—in the neighborhood of 10%—of developing incontinence afterward. Because of this similar range for all treatments, the issue of incontinence should not sway your treatment decision one way or the other. Obviously, there are some differences: patients are more prone to irritative symptoms from radiation and more apt to develop SUI from surgery.

A Patient's Story: Urinary Incontinence

Dwight W. is a 58-year-old African-American man. His father and first cousin had been treated for prostate cancer, so Dwight came to the office annually for a prostate exam and PSA. In 1 year, his prostate nearly tripled in size and his PSA jumped from 3.8 to 6.2 ng/mL. Although his prostate felt normal but slightly enlarged, it was obvious something was wrong. He reported that his urinary stream was weak and that he awoke every 3 hours during the night to urinate. A biopsy was done that showed a Gleason's 7 tumor that took up 40% of his prostate. He underwent a robotic prostatectomy, and when the urinary catheter was removed 1 week later, he was advised to begin pelvic floor exercises.

One month after surgery, he had total incontinence. As a bus driver in New York City, continence was necessary to keep his job. He feared not being able to return to work and became depressed. He admitted that he was not doing the exercises as he expected to return to normal without any effort, like his cousin had. What had happened was that his enlarged prostate had been causing him urinary problems before surgery, and because of its size, his prostate might have been doing more of the work holding the urine in than a normally sized prostate would, which may have caused his sphincter muscle to atrophy. His doctor encouraged Dwight to do the exercises as often as possible, several times every day. Two months later, his urinary control was about 90%, and 2 months after that, he no longer needed to use pads and was able to return to his regular work activity.

6

Treatments for Urinary Incontinence

For most men, the concept of being incontinent is a foreign and frightening one. You have already gone through the stress of having a cancer diagnosis and treatment, now you are faced with having to wear a pad in your underwear for fear of urine leakage. Urinary incontinence (UI), erectile dysfunction (ED), and bowel problems are three issues that most adversely affect the daily lives of men after prostate cancer treatment. For your physical and mental health, it is important to pursue therapy to address these embarrassing problems. Almost every patient can see at least some improvement in these side effects if he works with his doctors to find the best treatments for his particular difficulties.

As noted in the previous chapter, UI can manifest as either stress urinary incontinence (SUI) or urge urinary incontinence (UUI). The problem of SUI after surgery is the most common form and can affect men in varying degrees. The problem can vary from a squirt of as little as a few drops of urine with a strong sneeze when the bladder is full to a constant drip of urine. When incontinence is nearly constant (whether urge or stress), it is called total incontinence. Whatever the situation, a good first line of defense is to strengthen your equipment with pelvic floor exercises.

PELVIC FLOOR EXERCISES: AN EASY, NONINVASIVE TREATMENT FOR INCONTINENCE

Because SUI results from injury to the urinary sphincter, the first line of therapy for most men is to increase the strength of that muscle through exercise. If you exercise a muscle by lifting weights, the muscle will get larger. The same is true for the urinary sphincter. In this case, the exercise is not done by lifting barbells but by a conscious contraction of the muscle. The good news is that the exercises work and the reward will be dry underwear and less worry—if they are done religiously. Men can begin the exercises (usually called Kegels exercises) while waiting for surgery. As in Dwight W.'s case (cited in Chapter 5), many men are not motivated to do the exercises until they begin having incontinence after surgery. The fear of remaining in that condition provided the impetus for Dwight to do what had

> *"What one piece of advice would I give to those reading this book? Do your Kegels! I didn't do mine and I still go through two or three pads a day [more than a year after prostatectomy]."*
>
> —*Jake T.*

been suggested pre-operatively. You can begin Kegel exercises any time, although I do not recommend the exercise while the catheter is in place immediately after surgery. But you can begin again as soon as the catheter is removed.

The easiest way to contract the muscle is to stop urinating when the stream is going full blast. Remember that exercise is similar to lifting weights. The more weight (the heavier the stream you stopped), the greater the strength of the muscle, and the thicker it will become. It is this muscle thickness that will control the leaks of urine. It is important, even when control is obtained, to *continue* to do the exercise, as the muscle can revert to its prior weak state over time, especially as you grow older.

Another method to strengthen the urinary sphincter muscle is to contract the pelvic floor. In those exercises, the entire pelvic floor is contracted—that is, the urinary sphincter and the rectal sphincter. So the method is to contract the rectal sphincter multiple times. With each contraction of the rectal sphincter muscle, the urinary sphincter will contract too, and together they become stronger. Pelvic floor strengthening can also begin before surgery. In fact, increasing pelvic floor strength has been shown to reduce incontinence by more than 50% 1 year after surgery.[1,2]

If you find you are having difficulty learning how to do pelvic floor exercises, it is sometimes helpful to have place the tip of your finger in or near the anus and contract the muscles (doing this once is usually enough!). You will be able to feel the contraction so you will know you are doing it correctly. Keep in mind you can do this exercise at any time or place. This exercise is undetectable to the outside eye, as long as you have clothes on—and even naked, as long as no one's looking too closely—so you can do it anywhere. Some men aim for 50, 100, or 200 repetitions a day, done every time they stop at a red light, or wait for an elevator. Others combine pelvic floor exercises with deep breathing or meditation exercises, so that they feel calmer as they get stronger. Some doctors advocate more elaborate biofeedback methods with expensive machinery, but over time the results are no better than the self-directed pelvic floor exercises that can be done anywhere and anytime. The more they are done, the stronger the muscles will be and the less likely you will be to have serious incontinence post-treatment.

PURSUING FURTHER TREATMENT FOR URINARY INCONTINENCE

Pelvic floor exercises can be done before and after treatment to alleviate symptoms of incontinence, but they may not be enough on their own to treat more serious cases. The problem of stress incontinence is directly related to the strength of the urinary sphincter. If the nerves around the sphincter muscles are seriously injured, then the man will not be able to exert sufficient pressure to keep urine from leaking through it when the bladder fills. If the magnitude of the injury to the sphincter or the surrounding tissues and nerves is too great, then the pelvic floor exercises will not work. In those cases, the individual patient, with the aid of his physician, has to decide how aggressively he wants to pursue therapy and which therapy to use, as determined by his medical condition and his cancer status. Another important factor in deciding which therapy to choose is how long it has been since the prostate cancer treatment—the sooner, the better.

The concept of "bother" will help people make the decision about when and how to treat this side effect. Ask yourself the question, "How much am I bothered by my level of incontinence?" The answer may be different for different people; only you as an individual can make the decision. You might hardly be bothered by leaking urine—maybe because you have a very mild case of UI, or you have more interesting activities to focus on, or because you have more serious health problems to worry about. Or you might be terribly distraught and angry about incontinence. Or you may experience emotions somewhere between the two extremes. It is your degree of bother that should guide you and your doctor when deciding how aggressively to treat the problem.

Your doctor will have a general sense of your degree of incontinence by how many pads you go through in a day, but that is not always related to the degree of "bother" experienced. In one study, it was noted that of men who used one pad per day, 98% considered themselves continent—that is, they were satisfied with the result.[3] Men who require two or more pads per day are usually more adversely affected. In my urology practice, I have seen patients who were disappointed about the fact that they were leaking urine but had learned to live with the problem and were totally uninterested in any form of treatment. These patients typically learned what sorts of circumstances might be more likely to cause an incontinent moment and did what they could to avoid them. They accustomed themselves to wearing protective pads or undergarments and keeping themselves clean. Other patients have been terribly distraught over leaking even a few drops of urine during the day and vigorously pursue all avenues for improvement.

Most patients who suffer from incontinence fall somewhere in the middle—and each individual must decide for himself how long and how aggressively to treat this problem. If you do end up with some incontinence as a result of your cancer treatment, the important thing is to face your situation head-on and realize that there is no magic wand to wave that will restore you to your pretreatment state. It is up to you to decide just how much "bother" your level of incontinence causes and to be honest with your doctors and persistent if you do not immediately get the help you desire.

PHARMACEUTICAL TREATMENTS

In the discussion of Viagra and similar drugs in Chapter 4, it was made clear that most people prefer to take a pill to solve their medical problems. For many men, phosphodiesterase (PDE)-5 inhibitor drugs are a "magic pill" that solves their ED. Unfortunately there is no parallel drug for UI. However, depending on the type of UI you have, you may find considerable relief with drug therapies.

Urge Incontinence and Overactive Bladder Treatment

As mentioned in the previous chapter, overactive bladder (OAB) can be caused by radiation damage to the bladder area. It can also be "unmasked" by surgery—meaning that bladder problems existed before the prostatectomy, but the prostate was blocking the urine leakage; once the prostate is removed, the bladder overactivity becomes clear. No matter what the cause of the OAB, whether it is the sole problem or is experienced along with stress leaking, the initial treatment is done with oral medication.

The treatments used to treat overactive bladder include a group of medications known as anti-cholinergic agents. These drugs work by blocking the effect of acetylcholine, a neurotransmitter that is released by the nerves in the bladder wall, causing the bladder muscles to contract. If a medication interrupts the nerve signal, the contraction is blocked, and the bladder overactivity can be minimized or stopped. Anticholinergics such as Detrol LA, Enablex, Ditropan, Oxybutynin, or Vesicare are widely prescribed for the treatment of UUI.

Unfortunately, that same neurotransmitter is released by nerves to important organs all over the body. The problem with the drugs is their lack of effectiveness (one study found only a slight difference between anti-cholinergic drugs and placebo or no treatment)[4] and the large list of significant side effects. The side effects arise because the drugs work on cells elsewhere in the body, causing reactions such as dry eyes, dry mouth, headache, constipation, rapid heart rate, confusion, and forgetfulness with a possible worsening of mental function, particularly in older people with dementia, such as those with Alzheimer's disease. In rare cases, anti-cholinergics may worsen glaucoma and should not be used in patients who have glaucoma. That said, if you have OAB, it is worth trying one of these drugs to control the symptoms. If one drug doesn't work, others can be tried and the doses of the drug can be adjusted to maximize the effect or until the side effects become too bothersome. If you reach that point, then you stop taking them and begin looking to other treatment options.

If the drugs do not reduce the symptoms of OAB, the next option for UUI or OAB is intermittent injections of Botox into the bladder wall. Botox is the brand name for Botulinum toxin—it is actually made from a toxic bacterium that poisons the nerves. Like a movie star's face that has been injected with Botox, the bladder wall will "freeze" when injected with this drug, stilling the spasms that cause urine leakage. After the injection, some people cannot urinate at all for a period of days to weeks (they must be catheterized during that time). The injections must be repeated about two times per year as the effect of each injection wears off.

Treatment for Urinary Obstruction

Some men have trouble with urination before they get prostate cancer: the cause of this is usually benign prostatic hyperplasia (BPH) (*see* page 5)—in other words, an enlarged prostate—which is blocking the path of the urine going through the urethra. Patients could also experience an enlarged prostate after either type of radiation treatment for prostate cancer. Usually an enlarged prostate can give a man feelings of fullness or difficulty urinating a strong stream. The typical treatment for this problem is medication.

Table 6.1. Common Alpha-Blockers and Their Side Effects

Brand name	Chemical name	Side effects
Flomax	Tamsulosin	Abnormal ejaculation, dizziness, headache, flu-like symptoms
Cardura	Doxazosin	Dizziness, fatigue, edema, shortness of breath, hypotension
Hytrin	Terazosin	Weakness, dizziness, hypotension, nasal congestion, impotence
Rapaflo	Silodosin	Decreased ejaculation, diarrhea, dizziness, stuffy nose
Uroxatrol	Alfuzosin	Dizziness, headache, nausea, dry mouth, hypotension, diarrhea

A family of drugs called alpha-blockers was initially approved by the FDA to treat high blood pressure. An Israeli urologist, Dr. Marco Caine, discovered they could also treat the symptoms of urine flow obstruction by the prostate. The drugs work by relaxing the smooth muscle cells of the prostate and urinary tract, opening more space and allowing the urine to flow more easily. Although the drugs also have some effect on the smooth muscles of the bladder neck, alpha-blockers are usually not an effective choice for men who have had their prostate removed.

Men who take the drugs can expect to have an increase in urinary flow that averages 10% to 20%.[5] Each of these drugs has side effects, and all can have

---

A Patient's Story: Medication for Urinary Incontinence

Darren N. underwent combination radiation treatment for his prostate cancer a few years ago and his current prostate-specific antigen (PSA) is almost 0. "The side effects are what I've been grappling with," says Darren. Since his prostate is still intact, he is very bothered by urinary obstruction. His physician prescribed a Flomax-like drug that works well for his urinary dysfunction, but it has turned his body into a living Catch-22. "When I take it, it makes me impotent. If I don't take it, I'm potent, but I can't urinate." Taking Viagra to get an erection gives him different side effects like headaches and vision problems. With an adjusted dose of just a quarter pill, Darren is able to have sex with his wife—if, of course, he skips his UI pill.

"My wife understands the medical issues and sometimes she accepts it and sometimes she doesn't," says Darren. He has considered other options but for now is hoping that a new therapy may be available soon to ease his symptoms.

---

an effect on the iris of the eye, known as floppy iris syndrome. The syndrome is not good for a satisfactory outcome after cataract surgery. If you are going to have cataract surgery, alert your physician, as he or she may choose a different medication.

NON-SURGICAL TREATMENTS

Cunningham Clamp

The least aggressive form of therapy for SUI is the Cunningham Clamp. The clamp is like a small clothespin with a soft lining of foam that physically clamps down on the urethra to ensure it closes all the way (*see* Figure 6.1). It comes in three sizes, depending on penile girth, and is worn externally, on the patient, to stop any urine from dribbling.

The clamp can be worn during the day when you are up and about. It needs to be released when you urinate and also every few hours to ensure that the blood flow to the penis is not impaired. At night when you are lying down, the clamp is usually not needed because incontinence is minimal to none when you are in a horizontal position. In most men, correct use of the Cunningham clamp with the correct size and tension does not cause pain. If it does cause pain, then that is a red flag for potential serious problems, and the clamp should be removed.

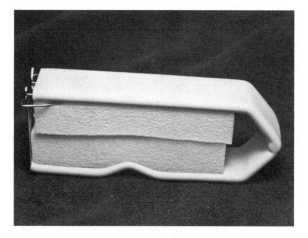

Figure 6.1 A Cunningham Clamp. The device is clamped around the penis and the pressure prevents urine from escaping. It needs to be released at intervals of several hours to allow urination and blood flow into the penis.

Condom Catheters

The next step up in degree of intervention is an external catheter—a condom-type device that is placed over the penis and secured in place to collect any urine that leaks out (*see* Figure 6.2). Originally the devices were made from actual condoms and the closed end was attached to a tube for drainage. Today they are specially designed and manufactured by medical supply companies. Because they are considered medical devices (as is the Cunningham clamp), Medicare Part B will pay for it if your doctor writes a prescription for you (make sure it is written to include all the parts such as leg bag, sealant, and leg straps).

To apply a condom catheter, several steps must be followed. Before the device is used, the hair at the base of the penis must be shaved or it will interfere with placement. After a daily washing of the penis and scrotum, you must blot-dry the skin and apply a polymer sealant to the skin of the penis where the condom will go. The sealant protects the skin from urine and allows the condom to be pulled off easily when the condom is changed. The condom has to be placed tight enough to maintain a leak-free environment but loose enough so as not to cause pain. The tightness is controlled by its size. To ensure a good fit, the catheter comes in five sizes (a size guide can be printed out from the manufacturer's website). The condom part of the device is usually changed daily and you can empty the bag when you wish. Obviously, the rate of filling of the bag depends

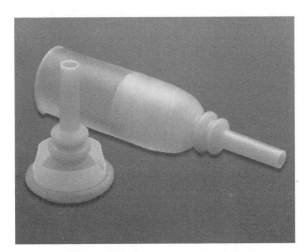

Figure 6.2 The Hollister external condom catheter. On the left is an unrolled catheter. The cylinder is placed over the penis, unrolled, and secured in place. The tube is connected to a bag worn on the leg.
(Courtesy of Hollister Incorporated, Libertyville, Illinois.)

on how much fluid you drink. The more liquids, the more urine you will make and the faster the filling of the collection bag. This collection bag is easily emptied into the toilet by opening a valve at the bottom of the bag.

The advantages of condom catheters include safety: it allows for cleanliness without surgery. By avoiding a long-term indwelling catheter, the risk of a painful infection in the bladder or kidneys is reduced. The price of using the external condom is constant vigilance that it is not leaking—and the odor that usually goes along with the wearing of the urine container strapped around your leg.

All in all, this is a safe and reliable method of treating incontinence, but it does require a commitment from the patient to keep himself clean and dry.

Indwelling Catheter

In rare cases, if the incontinence is particularly severe, an indwelling bladder catheter can be used temporarily. Like the condom catheter, it is also attached to a leg collection bag. The term *indwelling* means that the catheter is actually threaded up through the urethra (via the eye of the penis) and into the interior of the bladder. This is the same sort of catheter a patient gets after surgery or a hospital stay.

A PATIENT'S STORY: CONDOM CATHETERS

Eugene D. was an engineer in his late 60s who went to his doctor because he was troubled by urinary frequency. His doctor found prostate cancer, and Eugene elected to have radiation treatment: first seeds, then external beam therapy. His PSA returned to 0.0 ng/mL and he was cancer-free, but 6 months after the radiation, he began leaking urine almost constantly. It appeared that the radiation had damaged his urethra and urinary sphincter. The incontinence got worse and worse—Eugene's doctor sent him to a surgeon to explore the possibility of an artificial urinary sphincter, but the surgeon "had the bedside manner of a taxicab driver," so Eugene left and hasn't gone back. Instead, he bought a condom catheter at a pharmacy and wears the leg collection bag constantly. When the bag fills with a quarter-cup of urine, Eugene empties it into the toilet, sometimes as often as five or six times a day, for more than 3 years. "I think I've got a lot of patience—a lot of other people would've done something drastic by now." When we last spoke, Eugene had an appointment with another surgeon and was seriously considering further treatment. "I'm not afraid of death," says Eugene, "but if I'm going to live, I want to be able to live in some kind of comfort."

This system will ensure dryness, but at a price. First, wearing the catheter is uncomfortable (and sometimes outright painful), particularly during movement. Any catheter that is in place in the bladder for more than a few days almost always results in a urinary infection, as the bacteria migrate along the catheter into the bladder where they reproduce and grow. If the infection is from harmful bacteria, the infection can spread to other areas such as the testes or urethra or even the kidneys. Bladder stones can form as well. Therefore, long-term (i.e., months) use of a catheter is not a good idea. The other problem with using a catheter to keep you dry is that it will keep you from doing pelvic floor exercises. They cannot be comfortably done while wearing a catheter, so the man with a catheter is dry, but his muscles are weak. I try to restrict the use of a catheter after surgery to men who cannot afford to have an incontinence problem for a week or two because of some social or work obligation. Otherwise I try to encourage my patients to increase the level of pelvic floor exercise for at least a year after the surgery.

SURGICAL TREATMENTS

Although most men who have been through a prostatectomy are in no hurry to return to the operating room (and men who have had radiation are hoping to avoid it all together), sometimes surgery can offer the best, most permanent, treatment for incontinence. There are several surgical options for incontinence problems. The gold standard is an artificial urinary sphincter (AUS), but that is not the right choice for every patient. Alternatives to AUS are passive devices and bulking agents.

Bulking Agents

There has been some effort in the medical community to use bulking agents as a means to control SUI. A bulking agent is a paste-like substance that is injected just under the urethra, between the bladder neck and the urinary sphincter, to obstruct the flow of urine with sitting, standing, coughing, or any motion that makes you leak urine. The bulk of the paste causes increased resistance and reduces the leak. The substances that have been used for bulking paste include collagen, Teflon, silicone, body fat, cartilage cells, hyaluronic acid called Deflux, a combination of a water-soluble gel and silicone fibers called Macroplastique, and carbon microspheres called Durasphere. The most commonly used agent is a collagen-based product (Contigen).

The short-term result of the injection is reasonably effective, but the long-term result (longer than 6 months) is not good.[6,7] The injection is usually done in an operating room under anesthesia. This treatment can be used for men or women. For men, the problem is that after prostate cancer surgery or radiation, there is a good deal of scar tissue and it can be difficult to inject the product exactly to create the obstruction. Furthermore, the body absorbs collagen over time, so the injections need to be repeated about every year. Therefore, depending on the amount of scarring and the duration of the incontinence, it is not always a good option for treating SUI after prostate cancer therapy.

Another product, Durasphere, uses special silicone-covered beads to accomplish the same goal. It is permanent when injected, but for the same reason (scarring in the urethral area) can be difficult to place so that it is effective. The fat and cartilage-based pastes also get re-absorbed and usually require re-injection usually at least twice a year. Inflammation, scarring, and infection are all side effects of bulking agents.

Passive Devices

Similarly to the active urinary sphincter muscle, a passive device provides compression of the urethra, increasing the resistance to urine leakage from the bladder. It is the same as squeezing a hose that has a slow leak: the pressure on the outside of the hose will keep the water from dripping out.

Predecessor to Modern Passive Devices

The first modern surgical method used to control urinary leakage after prostatectomy relied on this concept of passive compression. Prior to the invention of silicone, natural body parts were modified to apply the pressure. The most logical choice was to use parts of the muscle that run alongside the penis, called the ischiocavernosus muscle. Its original purpose was to help stabilize the penis when erect and help maintain the erection by tensing and keeping the genitals filled with blood. The muscle is, like the appendix, no longer needed. A man can voluntarily contract his ischiocavernosus muscle. When this is done during erection, more blood is pushed into the end of the penis, and it will become slightly more erect but not enough to make a difference in most men. Some urologists long ago took the ends of the ischiocavernosus muscle, released them from their attachments, and crossed them over the urethra to the other side, thereby compressing the urethra. Although a novel idea, the muscle atrophied (got thinner) with time and the method did not prove successful. Today's methods are more sophisticated and more effective.

The same company that used silicone to create the first successful penile prosthetic implants, with the help of Joe Kaufman (my former chairman of Urology at UCLA), developed a series of urethral compression "pillows" to control urinary incontinence. The "pillows" were tied into place over the fattest portion of the urethra in the perineum—the area between the scrotum and anus—that passively put pressure on the urethra to keep the urine from leaking out. The long-term (5-year) results of that device were pretty good: about 70% of the men achieved continence without leakage. The placement required an operation and the complications included infection, the gradual erosion of the pillow, and lack of effectiveness either immediately or over time. The Kaufman prosthesis was used for about 10 years until the development of the AUS in the late 1970s. From that time until the present, the AUS has been the best surgical correction of SUI. However, the two companies that manufacture UI prostheses have recently introduced a new generation of passive sphincters or male slings in the style of the Kaufman device.

New Passive Devices

The reasoning behind the return to passive devices (also called male slings) is that many men have only a small amount of leaking that may be controlled with passive pressure on the urethra without the need to have to squeeze a pump in the scrotum each time he wants to urinate—an objection of many men to the AUS (*see* page 109). Men who have total or severe incontinence or leakage as a consequence of OAB are not candidates for the passive devices. There are three new pieces of equipment in this category: the InVance, the Advance, and the Virtue. Each of the devices is made of a man-made material that is surgically inserted against the urethra in the perineum (the area between the scrotum and the anus).

Both the InVance and Advance devices are similar in that they are made of an artificial mesh-like material that is surgically inserted against the urethra to compress it. The difference in the device is in the method of placement. The InVance, shown in Figure 6.3, is attached to the pelvic bone with permanent anchors. The AdVance is held in place through a process of pulling a special extension of the mesh through the pelvis. The mesh allows the in-growth of tissue into the spaces and the mesh plus the new tissue.

The proposed method of action is somewhat different for the Advance than in the passive-compression slings. In the Advance's case, the first portion of the urethra is dissected by the surgeon to allow the mesh to reposition the urethra up to 2 inches as a new way of enhancing continence. That repositioning effectively increases the functional length of the urethra to improve continence: the longer the urethral length, the greater resistance to outflow and the less leakage.

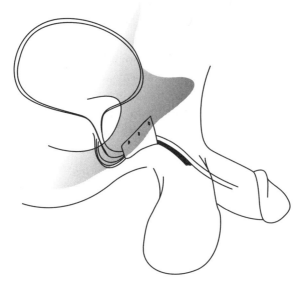

Figure 6.3 A diagram of the InVance® passive mesh device that compresses the urethra to prevent SUI of lesser amounts. The mesh in this device is fastened to the bony pelvis to support the urethra.
(Courtesy of American Medical Systems ®, Inc. Minnetonka, Minnesota; www. americanmedicalsystems.com.)

The overall success rate of the procedure (cured or improved) was 50% in one study and up to 70% in another. In comparison, the Invance's success rate at 2 years was reported to be about 74%.[8,9,10,11] Each follow-up was relatively short-term (less than 3 years), as the prosthesis has only been in use for a few years. The Virtue is also a sling device (*see* Figure 6.4), one that has just been introduced on the market so there are virtually no data to report about outcome with its use.

The complication rate is very low with these passive devices, with just a small number of men requiring an indwelling bladder catheter for a few days. There is minimal pain and the infection and erosion rates seem to be minimal.

Artificial Urinary Sphincter

The AUS is just that: an artificial replacement for the urinary sphincter muscle that is inserted permanently in the body and controlled by a pump you can manipulate at will. The earliest version of the AUS was introduced in 1972. The concept

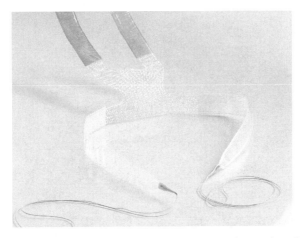

Figure 6.4 The Virtue® system, a passive mesh sling device designed to elevate the urethra to prevent SUI.
(Reprinted with permission from Coloplast, Inc.)

was a surgically placed silicone-based prosthesis that would not be rejected by the body, be long-lasting, and control total or stress urinary incontinence. The AUS has been upgraded through the years but its principal components are the same.

The AUS is composed of three parts, shown in Figure 6.5:

1. A pressure-regulating balloon in the bladder
2. A cuff that surrounds the urethra at point near the base of the penis
3. A pump in the scrotum.

The device is a closed hydraulic system filled with salt water. The pressure-regulating balloon delivers a constant pressure to the urethral cuff through the simple means of water pressure. That pressure expands the cuff, which in turn compresses the urethra, cutting off the urine flow. The pump can be controlled by squeezing the scrotum, which forces fluid up and out of the cuff, back to the balloon, releasing the pressure around the urethra.

When the man wants to urinate, he squeezes the pump several times, pushing pressure out of the cuff (see Figure 6.6).

When the cuff is deflated, the man can easily urinate. After he is done urinating, it takes about 90 seconds for the cuff to refill with fluid from the balloon, ensuring that urinary continence is regained. It is a brilliant system and the success rate for achieving total urinary continence with the AUS in most published series has been in the 80% range.

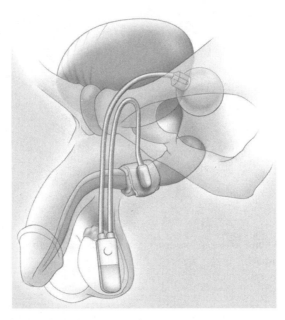

Figure 6.5 A diagram of the artificial urinary sphincter in position in the body.
The pressured balloon forces fluid (saline) at constant pressure into the cuff that wraps
around the urethra, keeping it closed and preventing urinary leakage unless the bladder
pressure exceeds the urethral pressure, as can occur during a cough with a full bladder.
(AMS 800®. Courtesy of American Medical Systems ®, Inc. Minnetonka, Minnesota;
www.americanmedicalsystems.com.)

Occasionally, if the pressure in the bladder is very high (e.g., during a violent
cough), then that pressure may overcome the resistance of the cuff and allow a
small leakage.

The AUS is inserted under anesthesia in the operating room by a urologist.
The patient is placed legs-up in the lithotomy position and an incision is made
through the scrotum to place the cuff and the pump. After the urethra is
exposed, a short segment (about half an inch) is isolated and measured for
properly sized urethral cuff (which comes in several circumferences, 3.5–6 cm).
After it is sized, the cuff is carefully placed around the urethra by the surgeon.
The cuff is attached to the pump, which is implanted in either the right or left
testicle (depending on whether the man is right- or left-handed), and attached
to the regulating balloon. The balloon is made of silicone material that lasts
indefinitely and will not be rejected by the body. The surgeon places the regulating balloon through a separate incision in the abdomen, in front of the bladder.
Once all three components are in place, the surgeon tests the connections to

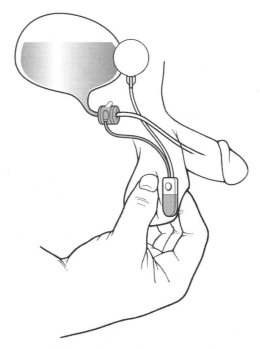

Figure 6.6 The position of the scrotal pump that is squeezed to empty the urethral cuff to allow the man to urinate.
(Courtesy of American Medical Systems ®, Inc. Minnetonka, Minnesota; www.americanmedicalsystems.com.)

make sure they work before closing the incision. The operation is quite simple and is done in less than an hour.

At the end of the surgery, the surgeon disables the pump, with the cuff in the open position, which allows the area to heal. It takes several days to a few weeks to recover from the surgery, but 6 weeks is the norm. During those 6 weeks, the man will continue to be incontinent and must use pads as before the surgery. At the 6-week post-operative visit, the surgeon will activate the pump by squeezing the testicle, and the cycling between the reservoir and the cuff begins.

In the early 1990s, some surgeons suggested that the overall continence rate could be increased by adding a second cuff to the system. However, in a recent published comparison of single- and double-cuff systems, there was no statistical difference in the number of pads needed after surgery in men with one or two cuffs (about 1.2 pads per day—down from nearly 8 per day), and there was a greater chance of post-operative problems with the double cuff.[12] The rates for complications are shown below:

Table 6.2. COMPLICATIONS FROM ARTIFICIAL URINARY SPHINCTERS

Complication	Single cuff (Number affected out of 25 men)	Double cuff (Number affected out of 22 men)
Erosion	2	2
Infection	2	2
Tubing leak	2	2
Atrophy	1	3
Mechanical failure	0	1
Urethral stricture	0	1
Fistula	0	1
Total	7	12

The best thing about an AUS is that you can regain continence in a short period of time and appear perfectly "normal"—no pads, no catheter—from the outside. The AUS also has good longevity. There are a few long-term follow-up reports that show a 10-year overall continence rate of 75% to 84%.[13,14] I have had some patients who begin to leak again 15 years after placement of the first AUS. This occurs because of thinning of the urethra in the area under the compressing cuff and requires surgical replacement of a new cuff around a new segment of the urethra.

The downside of the AUS is the possibility of infection during surgery and occasionally continued leakage if the pressure on the urethra is not complete. Also the patient must have the ability and willingness to squeeze the pump at regular intervals. Men with decreased strength in the hands (as after a stroke) or obesity—which makes it difficult to reach the pump—are not good candidates for AUS and may be better suited for the passive devices, even though those have a lower continence rate. Some men object to having to "pump"

A PATIENT'S STORY: ARTIFICIAL URINARY SPHINCTER

Walter R. was about 60 years old when he was diagnosed with prostate cancer. He elected to have a perineal prostatectomy, and was troubled by both ED and UI afterward. He had difficulty treating his ED, but luckily his incontinence has been well-controlled after getting an AUS. "It was a relief to have control back," Walter said. After just one night in the hospital, he had many years of relief before his first AUS wore out. He recently got a second AUS and although he now has to wear a pad for an occasional leak after a sneeze, he is largely satisfied by the outcome of his treatment and the ease of using an AUS: "Just press the right testicle to release the urine and that's it."

themselves to urinate, but others find it a small price to pay to have their continence restored. Again, the concept of "bother" can be your guide. Which is more bothersome: Your current level of incontinence or the need to pump out your urine? Obviously, neither is fun, but medical decisions often come down to choosing the lesser of two evils.

Finally, men who have an AUS and later require a bladder catheter for any reason (say, for heart surgery) must tell the physician that they have the device in place. It is possible to injure the urethra and damage the prosthesis if the physician is not forewarned.

A PATIENT'S STORY: ARTIFICIAL URINARY SPHINCTER

Frank S. was only 49 years old when he was diagnosed with prostate cancer. He had gotten a physical in preparation for running a marathon when his doctor accidentally checked Frank's PSA, thinking he was 50 years old and not 49. Frank's PSA came back as 54. An immediate biopsy was done and showed that about 80% of his prostate had been taken over by a tumor, and the cancer had already spread to the bladder wall and seminal vesicles. A veteran of the Vietnam War, Frank believes Agent Orange is probably to blame for his cancer. Luckily, he and his medical team were able to act quickly to save his life. Aggressive treatment was necessary and Frank quickly underwent surgery, followed by 40 doses of external beam radiation. Afterward, he had terrible problems with incontinence that just seemed to get worse over time. A few years later, he underwent surgery again, this time to get an AUS placed. "I'm glad I had it done, I really am. I still wear a small pad, but I'm good about 98% of the time."

MAKING A URINARY INCONTINENCE TREATMENT CHOICE

One recent study questioned whether, given the choice, patients would choose passive devices or artificial urinary sphincters to treat their incontinence.[15] The bottom line was that most men chose what was recommended by the surgeon who was guiding them. Of men who were recommended to have an AUS, 75% accepted that choice, whereas 100% of men who were recommended to have this sling chose to do so. Given the option of either, 92% chose the sling, which is the simpler operation.

Basically, the choice should be made based on the level of incontinence experienced. This can be measured in the number of pads needed per day for dryness. If more than six pads are required per day, I would say the AUS is the absolute choice. For less than three pads per day, the success with slings is about 67%; for three to six pads, the success rate is about 50%. Although there is not an extensive literature to rely on for data, it is possible that if the sling does not give a satisfactory result, then an AUS can be placed a later time.

A Patient's Story: Artificial Urinary Sphincter

Dave H. was 49 years old when he was diagnosed with a Gleason's 8 cancer. A perineal prostatectomy was performed and the tumor was found to extend into the bladder neck. After he returned to having full urinary control, Dave had to undergo post-operative external beam radiation as well. His PSA went from a pre-operative 8.4 to undetectable and remained that way for about 6 years. At that point, he began to have rapidly increasing PSA and was placed on andro-gen deprivation (hormone) therapy with Lupron.

Ten years after surgery, he began noting increasing stress leakage of urine. He went from not having to use any protective pads to up to four per day. Dave was an avid sportsman who liked to spend long days outdoors and did not wish to take any chances in being seen wetting himself in public. The options were discussed, and he chose an AUS. The AUS has been in place for 5 years. He voids every 4 to 5 hours and is pad-free. At this time, he is still dealing with an increasing PSA, but urinary control is no longer among his worries.

7
—

Other Complications and Their Treatment

As we discuss the complications that occur less frequently after prostate cancer care, it is important to repeat that with the exception of erectile dysfunction (ED), more than 80% of men who have either surgery or radiation therapy for their prostate cancer live relatively normal lives after treatment. With that in mind, for those 20% of men who do have a problem—the most common of which is urinary incontinence (UI)—the harm of the complication can significantly affect their quality of life.

In this chapter, we will address the rarer side effects that can result from prostate cancer treatment. Among these difficulties are several that may result from radiation treatment, such as urinary retention and different rectal issues, and some that more commonly occur after surgery, such as Peyronie's disease and penile shortening.

URINARY RETENTION

A significant complication of permanent seed radiation (brachytherapy) and radical prostatectomy is the inability to urinate after the treatment; this is known as urinary retention. It is the true opposite of urinary incontinence.

Urinary retention happens in the short term when the prostate swells in response to the radiation delivered by the seeds. This type of retention tends to occur within 1 day of the seed insertion. There are several risk factors for developing this complication: having a large prostate (more than 50 g, about twice the average size) and experiencing more symptoms of urinary urgency, frequency, and difficulty urinating before seed implantation.[1] In the long term, urinary retention can occur after surgery because of scarring of the bladder opening (bladder neck contracture) or in the urethra (urethral stricture).

The reported range of occurrence for urinary retention varies from a low of 1.5% to a high of 43% of brachytherapy patients followed by different studies. Most commonly reported are numbers of men who develop retention that are less than 5%[2]—so about 1 in every 20 men who choose seed therapy could reasonably expect to develop this complication.

Treatment of Urinary Retention

The initial treatment for urinary retention is placement of a bladder catheter, which may be needed for as long as 6 months.[3] After the catheter is in place, treatment proceeds with various medications to relax the prostate tissue, such as alpha-blockers like Flomax, tamulosin, Rapaflow, Uroxatrol, and with a family of drugs called 5-alpha-reductase inhibitors that shrink the prostate, such as Proscar or Avodart.

Somewhere between 11% to 60% of men (depending on which study you read) who have urinary retention may need surgery to remove the prostate to relieve the blockage. Of course, there are additional risks to having prostate surgery after seed placement—key among them is UI. But the bottom line is that this condition needs to be treated: you run a high risk of dangerous infections with a catheter in your bladder, and the quicker you can restore urination, the better.

If the urinary retention occurs after prostatectomy, then the treatment would be that for bladder neck contracture or urethral stricture.

BOWEL DYSFUNCTION

Bowel dysfunction can arise after radiation but not surgery. Bowel problems occur because the front wall of the rectum is located next to the back wall of the prostate. The radiation delivered to treat the prostate cancer, with either brachytherapy (seeds) or external beam radiation, can irritate this sensitive area and create problems for the patient. The new intensity-modulated external beam radiotherapy for prostate cancer was developed to maximize the dose of radiation to the prostate while minimizing the dose of radiation to the rectum and anus—in hopes of curing the disease while minimizing these types of complications. Unfortunately, high doses of radiation are usually needed to kill the prostate cancer cells, and the delicate cells lining the rectum are more susceptible to the effects of the radiation than are the hardy prostate cells. The net result is an upset to the normal function of the rectum. The name given to the radiation effect is *radiation proctitis*. The ending *itis* means "inflammation of," and inflammation of the rectum is characterized by diarrhea, intermittent rectal bleeding, abdominal pain, mucous discharge, and sometimes constipation. Between 2% and 20% of men experience proctitis of some kind after radiation therapy.[4] Those functional rectal changes should be thought of as either acute (i.e., occurring just after treatment) or chronic (developing more than 6 months after treatment).

Acute Proctitis

Acute proctitis refers to bowel problems that begin right after radiation treatment and usually resolve spontaneously within 6 months' time (a year at the outside). Associated with the changes that occur after radiation, acute problems include diarrhea, intermittent rectal bleeding, rectal ulceration, abdominal pain, rectal mucous discharge, and sometimes constipation. Acute proctitis is seen in 34% of patients after brachytherapy[5] and 43% of patients after external beam radiation.[6] Diarrhea is the most common symptom by far. Luckily, it usually responds to conservative treatment such as steroids or antibiotics. Other acute symptoms that soon pass are mild rectal urgency and mild bleeding.

Chronic Proctitis

Chronic proctitis may occur after 6 months, or as long as 2 years, post-treatment. The symptoms of chronic radiation proctitis are rectal urgency, fecal incontinence, pain, rectal strictures, mucous discharge, and rectal bleeding. Those problems arise because radiation affects the walls of the rectum, causing a thinning of the lining of the rectal walls and blood vessel abnormalities. The necessary continued moving of the bowels further irritates the area. All these factors make radiation patients more prone to bleeding. Of the men who develop chronic bowel proctitis—about 17% of brachytherapy patients[7] and 21.8% of external beam radiation patients[8]—two-thirds of them suffer from rectal bleeding.

Degrees of Severity

Rectal complications are categorized into degrees of severity, scored 1 to 5. Fortunately, almost all rectal side effects of radiation treatment for prostate cancer are low-grade and easily managed (not necessarily comfortable, but manageable).

Table 7.1. Various Grades of Rectal Complications

Complication	Grade 1	Grade 2	Grade 3	Grade 4	Grade 5[a]
Proctitis	Rectal discomfort; no treatment needed	Symptoms do not interfere with daily life but require medical therapy	Stool incontinence interfering with daily life; surgical treatment needed	Life-threatening, (perforation) surgery needed	Death
Rectal pain	Mild; does not interfere with daily life	Moderate; need pain medications but does not interfere with daily life	Severe; need medication and does interfere with daily life	Disabling	-
Spasms	Mild	Moderate	Severe	Disabling	-
Hemorrhage (bleeding)	Mild; no treatment needed	Symptomatic and medical treatment or minor cauterization needed	Transfusion and operative; intervention needed	Life-threatening consequences; major intervention needed	Death

[a] Trotti A, Colevas AD, Setser A, Rusch V, Jaques D, Budach V, et al. CTCAE v3.0: development of a comprehensive grading system for the adverse effects of cancer treatment. *Semin Radiat Oncol* 2003; 13(3):176–181.

In most cases, chronic proctitis can be treated with modest medication and hygiene pads placed in the underwear if there is some leakage of blood or stool. The goal of the management of chronic radiation proctitis (particularly bleeding) is to control the bleeding and reduce the need for office or hospital visits.

The medical therapies include enema treatments utilizing the drug sulfasalazine, steroids, and short-chain fatty acid enemas—these are not very effective and have tended to be used less in recent years. More aggressive therapies have had increased use, including lasers to cauterize the bleeding tissues—a treatment that 65% of patients responded positively to after just two treatments.[9] These aggressive interventions are rarely needed, but the patient must be aware that they are possible when choosing radiation as the primary mode of treatment.

PEYRONIE'S DISEASE

Peyronie's Disease (PD) was named for the French physician François Gigot de la Peyronie, who first described the disease in 1734. Essentially a scar in the penis causes it to curve during an erection. This curving (PD) is estimated to be present in about 3% to 9% of the male population. The problem usually begins with pain in the penis, followed by the man feeling a lump in the penile shaft. Then he will note a curve—either up toward his abdomen, down toward the floor, or to the side—when he has an erection. Although there are very rare cases in which PD has regressed without treatment, PD is nearly always permanent if it is still present 12 to 18 months after surgery. The good news is there are treatments that can prove effective.

Causes of Peyronie's Disease

In non-prostate cancer-related cases, it is believed that PD is caused by trauma—if there is no obvious trauma, then it may be that sexual intercourse causes small injuries (over many years) to the thick lining of the erectile bodies, and in men who are more susceptible to scarring as a response to injury, a thick plaque of scar tissue develops. In men who have had prostatectomies, there is a more obvious, and less enjoyable, cause for the scar tissue.

When the penis fills with blood during sexual excitement, it normally stretches as it elongates and becomes erect. However, the scarred area of the penis is not as elastic as normal erectile tissue and cannot stretch—as a result, the normal penis elongates around the scarred area, causing a bend (*see* Figure 7.1). The bend is called a "chordee." Think of the bend in a rainbow or in a bow as it is being pulled taut to release an arrow—that shape is a chord, hence the word *chordee* to describe a similar shape in a bent penis. There may also be an inherited component to the disease, as there are some limited familial relationships in men with PD.

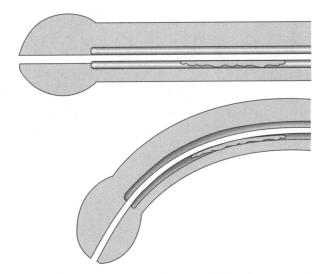

Figure 7.1 This illustration shows Peyronie's disease (PD) that can occur in men after prostate surgery. Because of the presence of a Foley catheter for at least a week and some urethral instrumentation during surgery, the lining of the inner surface of the urethra may become inflamed. In some men, the inflammation leads to the production of scar tissue around the urethra (shown as the light-colored area). Because scar tissue does not stretch, when the scarred penis becomes erect, the penis bends in the direction of the scar. The usual form of PD is found around the erectile tissue of the corpora cavernosa—not around the urethra. The urethral type is harder to treat. (Courtesy of Kelvin Davies, Ph.D.)

About 10% of men who have PD also develop scarring of the palms of the hands, in the crease just under the ring and little fingers, which if extensive will cause the ring and little fingers to permanently pull toward the palm of the hand. That disease is also named after a French physician; it is called Dupytren's Contracture, after Baron Guillaume Dupuytren, Napoleon Bonaparte's surgeon, who first described the condition.

Peyronie's disease after prostatectomy results from either accidental manipulation of the urethra with instruments during surgery or from having an indwelling urethral catheter for a number of days. Either the instrument or the catheter causes an inflammation of the urethral wall that extends into the base of the penis and causes scar tissue to develop (*see* Figure 7.1).

Men who are predisposed to scarring are probably more likely to develop that response. The scar may be small—less than half an inch long—or it may involve the entire penile shaft. Depending on the location of the scar, it may cause the penis to bend during erection, or, if there are equal amounts of scar on the top and the bottom of the penis, it may not cause the penis to bend. Some men (about 30% of those affected) do not even notice that they have PD.

Others who feel the lump of scar tissue immediately assume that it is a cancer and become very anxious. However, PD is very specific and is easily diagnosed by your urologist. *It never becomes a cancer.* The worst that PD can do is adversely affect your sex life and your psyche—but that is more than enough.

Post-operative PD is usually active for 12 to 18 months after surgery and then the inflammation stops. Unfortunately, by that time, the effect on the penis and erection are permanent for many men. There are a few reports of spontaneous return to normal with Peyronie's disease, but that occurrence is rare.

It is my experience in caring for men with PD after prostate cancer that they are often very angry about having the disease. Most surgeons do not tell their patients about the risk of PD before treating their prostate cancer, as it is a very uncommon side effect: there are no studies that have summarized the rate of PD after surgery, but based on my experience in practice caring for men with PD, I would estimate that 2% or 3% of prostatectomy patients develop some degree of PD. Patients tend to view its presence as another unexpected assault on their body, their masculinity, and their self-image. For some men, it is the last straw: "Why didn't he tell me that this could happen? I would not have gone ahead!" Other men find that they are unable to have sexual intercourse and PD takes a consequent toll on their relationships. Still others keep their PD in perspective: they don't like it, but they find that this cosmetic change in their body is less important to them than the fact that they are cured of cancer and may be completely continent, and perhaps even have normal rigid (but bent) erections. Frequently, men with PD suffer some degree of depression—if your negative feelings about your PD seem to be interfering with the activities of daily living, you might try some of the resources listed in the Appendix or Chapter 9.

Treating Peyronie's Disease

Of course, PD can be treated, but there are no established medical therapies that can be guaranteed to get rid of penile scar tissue and therefore cure the PD.

The medical treatment used by most urologists who care for PD patients is to inject the scar tissue with drugs that should reduce the plaque size. This is done through multiple injections—with a very small needle—directly into the scar tissue. The primary drug used is called Verapamil, a member of the family of drugs known as calcium channel blocking agents. Injecting the drug in high concentrations, directly into the plaque, should reduce the accumulation of collagen (which is the principal component of scar tissue), and over time the scar will disappear. It may take 6 weeks to a couple of years of injections to see results. (Luckily PD treatment is covered by most insurance.) In my experience, Verapamil injections work about 60% of the time. In some men, the scar is reduced, but the chordee remains. Other oral drugs have been used for the same purpose, such as Potaba, steroids, and colchicines, but none have passed rigorous scientific scrutiny as an effective cure. An injection of the drug collagenase is an enzyme that attacks collagen and therefore theoretically dissolve the plaque),–but it has not gained much popularity among urologists who specialize in treating the disease.

SURGERY FOR PEYRONIE'S DISEASE

If the chordee does not respond to injections, then, if the man (and his partner) desires, the penis can be straightened surgically. There are four types of surgery that are currently used to correct the chordee of PD. (None of them require insertion of a bladder catheter, which cuts down on the risk of further scarring.)

The simplest and least risky surgery is called the Nesbitt Plication. In this operation, the longer side of the penis is shortened to "even up" the penis so it is straight. The operation is done by placing suture material into the tough covering of the penis and creating a pleat, so that it shortens the length of the tissue on the normal side of the penis. Thus, the normally elastic tissue can no longer elongate and the longer normal side of the penis is now shortened, "evening out" the penis and preventing it from bending. The operation is very safe, cannot make problems worse, and can even be done under local anesthesia. Its principal drawback, of course, is that it shortens the penis. Nesbitt Plications tend to be done in men who have chordees less than 45 degrees (and some length to spare). If the bend is more severe than 45 degrees, then no one would want to lose enough penile length to make up for that big a bend.

If the curve is more than 45 degrees, then a tissue replacement operation needs to be done. There are two variations of this surgery: the scar is either cut into or removed and a piece of replacement tissue larger than that removed is used to fill the gap. The replacement tissue can be harvested from the patient, or other sources, and used to fill in the gap. I favor the use of the person's own tissue, usually a bit of dermis (the underlayer of skin) from the love handle area (so your waistline's whittled at the same time. . .). After this operation, it takes about 6 months for the skin graft to soften and become normal to the touch. However, it works most of the time and the men can have sex about 6 weeks after the surgery.

One of the problems in men who have PD after prostate cancer care is that the scar tends to form on the bottom of the penis and that area is not a good place to do scar excision surgery as it overlies the urethra. In that case, I recommend penile implant surgery to correct the problem, which is a good choice for men who are having ED as well as PD. A penile implant, either a semi-rigid or inflatable, will correct the chordee and correct any erectile dysfunction problems at the same time. (*See* pages 78–84 for more information about implants.) Because the implant straightens the penis, it is not necessary to remove or alter the scarred area of the penis.

A Patient's Story: Peyronie's Disease

Jake T.'s father died of prostate cancer at age 69, so Jake was vigilant about his annual PSA tests. By the time he reached age 57, Jake's PSA had crept up enough that his internist recommended a biopsy—a good thing, because the results showed cancer in three-fourths of his prostate. He consulted with several surgeons before choosing a very busy and successful doctor to perform his robotic prostatectomy. "Everybody minimized the risk of incontinence and no one even mentioned Peyronie's."

Jake's surgery successfully treated his cancer, but left him with temporary ED and UI and a bad case of Peyronie's disease. "I was so not prepared for the aftermath," says Jake. "I had no clue about the catheter—anything. I thought the whole damn thing stunk—the surgery, aftermath, and Peyronie's especially." Jake wonders if the catheter was the cause of his PD. "I can't bear—that's not true—I am acutely aware of my erection. It feels foreign to me now. My wife is very gracious and says she can't feel the difference when we're making love." As for Jake, "I try to remain present. I can feel it. I have some pain during intercourse. . . I love my penis. I've always had an active sex life. Now I'm working my way back to that." Jake is currently undergoing injections in hopes of straightening out his penis.

PENILE SHORTENING

Loss of penis length is a complication that can occur after a prostatectomy in which the nerves are not spared. The majority of prostatectomies are done in such a way as to spare the nerves that run down either side of the prostate; these are the nerves that send signals to the penis to become erect. Unfortunately, not every prostatectomy can spare the nerves because of the size or location of the tumor or the unique anatomy of the man (*see* pages 26 and 55 for a fuller discussion of nerve sparing).

It has been suggested by several researchers that those nerves going to the penis also help keep certain cells called smooth muscle cells alive. When the nerves are destroyed during surgery, the cells die. This accelerated death of the smooth muscle cells means that the cells are not replenished, and because the bulk of the penis is made up of smooth muscle cells, the penis loses volume.

This accelerated cell death, known as *apoptosis*, will occur if the nerve damage is caused by surgery or any type of radiation, high-intensity focused ultrasound (HIFU), or cryotherapy (*see* Chapter 11 for a description of these therapies). Some doctors propose using PDE-5 inhibitors (i.e., Viagra, Levitra, Cialis) to reduce the amount of apoptosis. However, studies have not given convincing evidence that they make a difference; thus, the claims are not yet substantiated by scientific evidence.

The second possible cause of penile shortening after erectile nerve damage is an increase of scar tissue in the penis' cavernous bodies resulting from damage during surgery or other treatments. In this case, the penis will be shortened—sometimes evenly, sometimes more to one side (in which case it is PD). Remedies for penile shortening resulting from scar tissue are similar to those for PD.

Rectal problems, urinary retention, PD, and penile shortening are not common complications from prostate cancer, but they can be traumatic problems for those who experience them. In the next chapter, we will turn to another topic that is also fairly rare in the modern world: more serious cases of prostate cancer and their treatment.

Non-Localized Cancer
Treatments and Complications

Of the nearly 218,000 American men diagnosed with prostate cancer in 2010,[1] about 90% had localized prostate cancer at the time of diagnosis, meaning cancer that had not spread outside the prostate. The other 10%, or about 21,800 men, already had cancer that was non-localized—that is, the tumor had spread outside of the prostate at the time of their diagnosis. Thanks to modern hormone therapy, the diagnosis of locally advanced prostate cancer is no longer an immediate death sentence and many fine years of fruitful life can be had. The vast majority (at least 85%) of patients with advanced cancer do respond to hormone therapy, which can transform the cancer into a chronic but manageable disease for years ahead. It cannot be predicted in advance who will respond, and who will not, or for how long the response will last in any one man. Some reports have shown that 25% of men who are placed on immediate hormone therapy will survive 10 years or longer.[2]

Like localized prostate cancer, the advanced form of the disease can also arrive with few or no symptoms. Luckily, the modern prostate-specific antigen (PSA) tests catch most prostate cancers before they metastasize. In the unfortunate event that your cancer is advanced at the time of diagnosis, you may have actually gone to the doctor because you had symptoms as vague as weakness or back pain. (Because the blood drainage from the prostate gland tends to go to the spinal column, that is one of the first places to which the prostate cancer may spread.) In most men with metastatic prostate cancer, they have an initial elevation of the PSA and not much else. Prior to the use of PSA for early diagnosis, 50% of the men had a first diagnosis of prostate cancer that was metastatic or non-localized. Even in the era of PSA, an occasional man will come to the office that has not had, or neglected to follow up on, an earlier medical exam or report, and finds that his cancer has already progressed.

DIAGNOSING NON-LOCALIZED PROSTATE CANCER

The best treatment for any man with prostate cancer is determined by the stage of the disease at diagnosis. Advanced prostate cancer is considered Stage 3 or 4. Your doctor determines the stage of your prostate cancer by using a combination of the size and location of the cancer and the Gleason's score (*see* pages 13–17 in Chapter 1). The stages of localized prostate cancers are Stage 1, a small area of cancer in one lobe of the prostate; or Stage 2, a cancer that may occupy one or both sides of the rostate. Non-localized prostate cancer stages are Stage 3a, which extends out of the prostate in one or both sides, and Stage 3b, which extends into the nearby seminal vesicles. Because they are the first organs invaded by prostate cancer, the seminal vesicles are usually removed during a standard prostatectomy. Stage 4 cancers extend into the local tissues other than the seminal vesicles, including the rectum, bladder neck, pelvic muscles, or external sphincter—or beyond. All recurrences of prostate cancer (i.e., prostate cancer that returns months or years after it has been treated and the PSA returned to 0.0 ng/mL) are by definition non-localized.

When the doctor first diagnoses you with prostate cancer, the cancer stage he gives you is called a "clinical stage." This means it is the stage of your cancer as best your doctor can determine through the clinical tools at his or her disposal. Those tools are the digital rectal exam, which allows the doctor to feel the tumor, your PSA scores (and past scores), magnetic resonance imaging (MRI) or other scans, and the Gleason's score, determined when the cells from your biopsy are analyzed by a pathologist. When you opt for surgical treatment, the stage of your cancer will be confirmed or revised, based on what the surgeon sees inside your body and what a pathologist may find when your surgically removed prostate is sent to the lab. A more precise idea of the cancer's aggressiveness is determined by examining cancer cells under a microscope from samples taken of the prostate. Most of the time, clinical stages are proven correct during this process, but patients should be aware that the clinical stage can under- or overestimate the actual state of the disease.

It is relatively easy to make the diagnosis of a Stage 4 tumor, but Stage 3 tumors are more difficult to accurately assess before treatment, even with an MRI or other scans. Stage 3 prostate cancer is best diagnosed after radical prostatectomy, when the entire prostate can be examined by the pathologist and the full extent of the tumor is determined under the microscope. As a result, about one-third of men who undergo prostatectomies are "upstaged" to Stage 3 after their prostatectomies, because the true microscopic extent of the disease

> *"My coping mechanism? I don't think about it. The only time it bothers me is when I have to go see Dr. Melman. For the next 3 months, I put it out of my mind."*
> —*Reggie M.*

is revealed in the lab. Not all of these men must have additional treatment, however. At times, the cancer is just barely out of the prostate capsule and has not yet invaded any other organ, and it is possible to remove all the cancer during surgery. If the tumors have spread to the bladder neck or seminal vesicles, then radiation and/or hormone therapy should be prescribed.

THE IMPORTANCE OF PSA TESTING AFTER PROSTATECTOMY

Many men are confused about the importance of their PSA test after prostatectomy. The issues are straightforward. If the prostate and the cancer are completely removed, then the PSA should be 0.0 within a few weeks after surgery (the time it takes to rid all the PSA from the blood), because there is nothing left to secrete PSA. If the PSA is not 0.0 ng/mL a few weeks after radical prostatectomy, then there is either a small amount of benign (non-cancerous) tissue left behind at the surgery site, or the cancer has spread—either to local tissue, or distant areas such as bone or lymph nodes—and is secreting small amounts of PSA into the bloodstream. Unfortunately, any spread to distant organs is microscopic in the early stages and cannot be pinpointed, even with the many methods available today. In other words, a man whose PSA is not 0.0 ng/mL after surgery may have a tiny bit of prostate cancer lurking just about anywhere in his body and his doctor will probably not be able to say how much cancer or where.

Whether or not a man's PSA returns to 0.0 ng/mL after treatment for localized prostatecancer, he will have to continue to have his PSA monitored for the rest of his life to ensure that the cancer does not return. At first, he will have to return for testing every 3 months. After 5 years with a 0.0 ng/mL PSA, the patient is considered cured but will still have to have PSA tests done annually for life. There are cases of recurrences that pop up 10 years or more after the first prostate cancer.

TREATMENT OPTIONS FOR ADVANCED PROSTATE CANCER

The reason that accurate staging is important is because the recommendation for treatment of the non-localized Stage 3 and Stage 4 cancers are different than those offered to men with localized tumors.

The treatment options to men with known Stage 3 cancer are:

- External beam radiation therapy plus hormone therapy
- Hormone therapy only
- Radical prostatectomy, which may be followed by radiation and/or hormone therapy depending on the pathology
- No treatment if another disease is present that may cause death first

Stage 4 cancers that have already spread to bladder, rectum, or lymph nodes or other more distant organs are not curable, but treatment can still slow or stop the growth of the cancer, relieve symptoms, or, at the very least, buy the patient some more time to live. The treatment options may include:

- Hormone therapy
- External beam radiation and hormone therapy
- Surgery to relieve symptoms of prostate obstruction

A PATIENT'S STORY: IMPORTANCE OF PSA FOLLOW-UP

John D. went to his family doctor because of sudden but constant leg weakness and pain. The doctor's work-up of John's condition showed a bone cancer known as multiple myeloma. However, the tests for that cancer proved negative. His PSA test was greater than 200 (more than 50 times normal), so John was sent to me for evaluation. I did a rectal examination and found that although his prostate was only mildly enlarged, one entire side was bony hard. A biopsy showed the presence of a Gleason's 9 tumor in all cores of his prostate. I asked if he had prior prostate exams. John admitted that his doctor had found an abnormal result on rectal examination 1 year earlier, in the presence of a slightly elevated PSA, and had suggested a urological consultation—but he hadn't followed up.

By the time he saw me, John had non-localized Stage 4 prostate cancer. I immediately placed him on androgen deprivation therapy (ADT) for pain relief and tumor control. He required orthopedic surgery to treat the bone cancer to prevent fracture of the hipbone that was weakened by the cancer. All these treatments used are employed to control the cancer and to maintain the best quality of life for as long as possible.

It is difficult to estimate how long men will respond to treatment if they have metastatic disease when they are first diagnosed, particularly if they respond to hormone therapy. A positive response (drop in PSA to 0.0 ng/mL) could add many years to their life. If the person does not respond (his PSA levels do not drop to near 0.0 ng/mL) then he has about a 50–50 chance of dying within 3 years of diagnosis from complications of the disease.

A Note on Stage 4 Prostate Cancer Treatment

When a cancer is Stage 4, meaning it has spread dramatically around the body, the treatment goal is typically supportive and not curative. This doesn't mean no treatment: indeed, a patient with Stage 4 may still undergo hormone therapy, chemotherapy, or radiation treatment, but these treatments are done to delay further decline, not to cure the cancer. We do stress that every patient should be treated, because it is impossible to know which men will respond successfully. Any one man may live for a long time—10 years or more—with Stage 4 cancer. Stage 4 patients must walk the tightrope between hope and realism: 80% of these patients die within 5 years of their diagnosis. However, that means 20% don't—and even those five years can be good ones. With help from a supportive medical team and family and friends, Stage 4 patients can still accomplish positive goals and improve their post-diagnosis health through appropriate treatment. *See* the Appendix for resources helpful to Stage 4 patients.

A PATIENT'S STORY: STAGE 4 DISEASE

Arthur Y., a 60-year-old man from West Africa who had lived in the United States for 15 years, had never had a PSA test or a digital rectal examination. His health was great, and he had no urinary symptoms. On examination, Arthur's prostate was firm but without nodules and of normal size for his age. His first PSA test was abnormally high, with a total PSA of 20 and a free PSA of 8%. Whenever I obtain a lab test that is unexpected, I repeat it to make certain that the test was not in error. A repeat PSA 1 week later showed the same numbers. The following week, I did a biopsy that showed Gleason's 8 tumors on both sides of Arthur's prostate. To help clarify which treatment would be best, I sent Arthur for a bone scan and a CAT scan. The bone scans showed evidence of cancer in his spine, which was confirmed on the CAT scan. The diagnosis was a metastatic prostate cancer with Stage 4 disease. Arthur began ADT (hormone therapy), and within 2 months his PSA fell to 0.0 ng/mL—a great result. He continued his normal life on that regimen and remains with a PSA of 0.0 ng/mL after 2 years of treatment.

Treating Non-Localized Prostate Cancer: Radiation Therapy

As mentioned above, some men are presumed to have a lower-stage, localized cancer until after their prostatectomy, when pathological evidence from the removed prostate—or a PSA score that does not drop to 0.0 ng/mL after removal of the prostate—indicates that the cancer may have already spread. Usually this means there is a microscopic amount of cancer elsewhere, but it could also be a microscopic amount of benign prostate gland remains. If your PSA does not return to 0.0 ng/mL after prostatectomy, and your medical team is not sure whether there is a metastasis and if so, where it is, then you have an important decision to make. One of two strategies can be followed:

1. Immediately and pro-actively treat the prostate bed with radiation, not really knowing if the tumor might be at a distant site and therefore not affected by the treatment
2. Do watchful waiting (carefully following PSA levels at frequent intervals) and augment with radiation therapy when the need becomes obvious (i.e., your PSA rises or new tumors begin to show up on scans). Doing radiation at this phase is known as "salvage" radiation.

An additional quandary exists if the post-operative pathology slides show that the cancer has extended outside of the prostate, but your post-operative PSA is still 0.0 ng/mL . (Obviously, the first action would be to retest your PSA to confirm the score.) That would mean either there are no more cells left behind and the cancer is cured *or* that there are so few cells left behind that the PSA they secrete cannot be measured—but those cells will multiply, the cancer will eventually progress, and the PSA will begin to rise. Again, you could have radiation immediately, but radiation does carry possible complications—urinary incontinence, erectile dysfunction (ED), and an increased risk of rectal symptoms, because the prostate gland itself is no longer blocking the rectum from some of the radiation beams. Or you could wait and see.

*A quick flash-back to junior high math class: the **median** is the score that is exactly in the middle—half the results are higher, half are lower. It is important to remember that a median can be different than the average (in which all the scores are added together and divided by the number of scores).*

In this case, where the PSA does return to 0.0 ng/mL after surgery but Stage 3 disease is diagnosed by pathology, published research shows that if not treated, the median time to measurable (by MRI or other scan) metastatic disease is 8 years. This seems like a fairly long time until you consider that the study also showed that the median time to death from the cancers was 5 years after that: a total median of 13 years from point zero to death.[3]

Not knowing whether the cancer is cured is a very stressful situation. Some men prefer to do radiation right away because it is something they can do and they prefer not to worry when the other shoe will drop. Others prefer to avoid any further treatment until absolutely necessary and wait until their PSA rises or other signs of continued cancer appear.

The Case for Immediate Radiation

In addition to the life-or-death stakes, the decision of what to do and when to do it has been difficult because research is slim in this area. A researcher may have to wait 15 years after a particular patient's treatment to understand how well that patient's treatment choices worked. Recently three research groups (one American and two European) addressed that issue and appear to have found the answer.[4,5,6] The studies followed patients for 15 years, from around age 65 up into their 80s. The goal of the these studies was to compare the outcome of two treatments for men who were discovered to have Stage 3 disease at the time of their surgery: either to give immediate external beam radiation or not to give radiation unless they developed a recurrence of the cancer, as measured by increase in the PSA. The conclusion from all three of the studies is that *immediate external beam radiotherapy (within 18 weeks after surgery, as soon as urinary control is regained) offers a survival advantage of about 10% over no radiation or delayed radiation.*

The studies also tracked how long these patients continued life with no evidence of disease—a complete cure—as the outcome (measured by no PSA recurrence). This is very important to prove that Stage 3 disease is not a death sentence. In a study of 211 men treated with observation only (no treatment), 97 men survived without metastatic disease. The median metastasis-free survival was 12.9 years—half survived even longer with no recurrence. Remember these are men in their 60s and 70s, most of whom probably would have lived a similar length of time if they had never gotten prostate cancer. In the same study, 214 men received immediate radiation treatment after surgery; 93 men survived with a metastasis-free survival of 14.7 years—an additional 2.5 years than those who had no treatment. The men who were treated tended to live longer without disease recurrence. The pre-operative PSA rate or Gleason's score made no difference to the cure rate. Even when the cancer had spread to the seminal vesicles in the surgical pathology specimen, thought to be a particularly dangerous finding, there was an improvement in 10-year overall survival from 51% to 71%, if the patients received immediate post-operative radiation.

The outcome is not quite as good if the PSA does not return to 0.0 ng/mL after surgery. But even in that event, at 10 years after post-surgery radiation, the metastasis-free survival for those patients is 73%, which is 8% higher than if no radiation is given. Similar results were obtained in a large European study, suggesting that the findings are real and believable.[7,8]

Is there a cost to the having the radiation? The answer is probably yes, but frustratingly, details are hard to come by and specific numbers are not available for comparison. The primary risk from the radiation is the worsening of erectile function. Nearly all men who have both surgery and radiation therapy will suffer from ED permanently post-treatment.

THE SALVAGE RADIATION OPTION

With that in mind, if you have a PSA of 0.0 ng/mL, but were diagnosed with Stage 3 cancer after surgery, then you might say, "What if I treasure my erections and sex life and want to wait to see if my PSA will rise before having radiation?" Radiation given in the presence of a rising PSA, more than 6 months after surgery, is known as "salvage" radiotherapy. The outcome of such salvage therapy was recently reported by a research group in Germany.[9] The possibility of a long-term (10 years post-treatment) cure—that is, PSA equal to 0.0 ng/mL—is only about 20 to 25% for those patients. In comparison, 73% of men given immediate radiation therapy enjoy a 0.0 ng/mL PSA 10 years after treatment.

Achieving a PSA of 0.0 ng/mL with salvage radiation therapy depends on at least two factors.

1. Having a low PSA after surgery but before salvage treatment is associated with having a better outcome with salvage radiation. A specific level has not been defined, but the *failure* rate for salvage radiation is only 37% if the PSA is less than 1 before salvage treatment. However, the *failure* rate jumps to 72% if the PSA is greater than 1 before salvage treatment.[10]

2. Whether the cancer had extended to the seminal vesicles already at the time of surgery and how low the stage of the cancer was at the time of surgery also both affect the success of salvage treatment (the lower the clinical stage at surgery, the better chance of positive outcome).

If the salvage radiation therapy was a success, then the patient's PSA will return to undetectable levels afterward. If it does return to undetectable, then that's great news—about 75% of those with undetectable PSAs still have no evidence of returning cancer after 8 years (as compared to about 15% of patients whose PSA did not drop to undetectable).[11] If the patient's PSA did not become undetectable, that means the tumor was either unresponsive to the radiation or, more likely, was at a site that was not reached by the radiation. When the PSA is low, and the cancer is at microscopic levels, it is impossible to diagnose cancer that lies outside the prostate bed.

So the treatment is a bit of a crapshoot: it may work, it may not work, and you will not know until after the treatment is given. The odds for longer life are clearly in the man's favor if he accepts the immediate radiation. (Hypothetically, there is a chance that a man's age and situation in life may make this argument less compelling to him.) However, the choice for radiation therapy must be made by the patient and his partner and depends on how important normal erections are for their quality of life, if the man is still potent. Remember that surgical- and radiation-induced ED can be treated with intra-cavernous injection therapy or penile implants (*see* Chapter 4) for those who wish to continue to have sexual intercourse and the potential for a longer disease-free life.

This choice of radiation is not a part of every patient's journey: most men with non-localized disease at the time of prostate cancer diagnosis (as opposed to post-surgically) face a different treatment, hormone therapy, which can bring other difficult choices and consequences into their lives.

Hormone Therapy for Non-Localized Prostate Cancer

Androgen deprivation therapy, or hormone therapy, is the most common form of treatment for non-localized prostate cancer. An androgen is any kind of hor-mone that controls male sexual development or processes—the most prevalent androgen is testosterone. Testosterone is the primary male sex hormone that helps men be "manly." It helps male sexual organs and secondary sexual char-acteristics (such as facial hair and a deeper voice) develop during puberty and plays a lifelong role in maintaining a man's muscles, energy, and libido. Testosterone is produced mainly in the testes but also in smaller amounts by the pituitary gland in the brain. Production declines naturally with age for most men, which can result in a lower sex drive, declining muscle mass, and a less frequent need to shave.

The goal of all ADT therapies is to lower the blood testosterone to the level of someone who has no testes production of the hormone. That can be accom-plished with surgical removal of the testis, or with chemical removal of the testosterone production using female hormones (estrogens), drugs that block the testosterone production like ketoconazole, drugs that affect the pituitary gland and stop its production of testosterone, and drugs that block the affect of testosterone on the prostate.

How Androgen Deprivation Therapy Works

Depriving the body of testosterone to control prostate cancer is a medical concept discovered about 70 years ago. In 1941, Charles B. Huggins, one of two urologists to ever receive a Nobel Prize in medicine, and his colleague Clarence V. Hodges, reported that prostate cancer was hormonally responsive and could be treated (i.e., controlled but not cured) by removing the hormone testosterone from the patient's bloodstream.[12] Back in that time, testosterone removal was accomplished by actual surgical castration or by doses of the female hormone estrogen, which causes the testes to stop making testosterone.

Most prostate cancer cells need testosterone for growth and maintenance. When testosterone is removed from the blood, it causes the early death (apoptosis or cell death) of most, but not all, the cancer cells. The cells that do not die may grow slowly over many years. In about 15% of the men with metastatic disease, the cancer cells are not responsive to testosterone withdrawal; they are called "castration-resistant" cells and continue to grow unabated until they cause the death of the person. However, for 85% of patients, removing the testosterone can greatly improve their cancer survival.

Androgen deprivation therapy is *not* chemotherapy, which is the treatment that many people receive to control other types of advanced or metastatic cancers. Chemotherapy uses toxic chemicals to block the growth and reproduction of many cells. Because testosterone has a specific relationship to prostate cancer, ADT is a primary therapy for men with metastatic or advanced disease at the time of prostate cancer diagnosis (as opposed to those who are "upstaged" to advanced disease post-surgery). That means that the cancer has spread to other places in the body and is not curable by surgery or radiation; therefore, controlling the growth of the tumor and reducing the symptoms caused by the tumor (such as bone pain or bladder obstruction) are the primary goals of treatment.

Basically, hormone therapy has made it possible for prostate cancer to become a chronic illness, kept in check with medication, like diabetes or high blood pressure. When a patient goes off his medication, the cancer will start right back up again. This is because the cells are starved out when testosterone is removed from the body, but once that hormone starts flowing again, the cancer has the fuel it needs to multiply. Unfortunately this means that patients with advanced prostate cancer have to stay on hormone therapy for the rest of their lives.

Sometimes ADT is used for localized disease as well. It is now used routinely, typically for a 3-year treatment, in men who have external beam radiation as their primary treatment for localized (Stage 1 or 2) prostate cancer. Adding 3 years of ADT (typically begun before the radiation and continuing afterward) to external beam treatment has improved the survival rate for these patients.[13]

In one study, 970 men were given either 6 months or 3 years of androgen suppression. The results showed only a slight survival advantage to the 3-year group. Side effects included hot flashes, reduced libido, and reduced sexual activity in both groups but were worse in the 3-year ADT group. In addition to controlling the cancer itself, ADT can also ease symptoms of advanced prostate cancer, such as bone pain, spinal compression, and urethral obstruction.

Kinds of Androgen Deprivation Therapy

For about 40 years after the Huggins report, the two methods most commonly used to achieve testosterone reduction were surgical castration (orchiectomy, the removal both testicles) or the administration of the female hormone estrogen. Each had their problems. Although castration was often effective for reducing the level of testosterone in the blood and controlling the growth of the tumor, it was (obviously) a hard sell to the patients. Also, testosterone is manufactured in the adrenal glands as well as the testes, so even after castration there was incomplete suppression of the cancer in some men. In theory, orchiectomies can still be used today as a lower cost alternative to ADT. In some parts of the world, this is the best treatment available.

The female hormone estrogen was given as a pill in a 5-mg/day dose. The effect of that dose of estrogen tricked the body into stopping production of a hormone called luteinizing hormone (LH). Luteinizing hormone is the hormone that drives the testes to manufacture and release testosterone. In a large study done in the 1970s, it was discovered that men with prostate cancer who were placed on 5-mg/day of estrogen had a higher death rate from stroke, blood clots, and heart attack than men who did not receive the drug. Lesser doses had fewer side effects but reduced effectiveness in controlling the cancer. Although the estrogen helped shrink the cancer, as a consequence of that study, estrogen therapy fell out of favor in the United States.

Fortunately in the 1980s, a new type of drug was invented to control cancer through hormone suppression. That drug is a long-acting product called *luteinizing hormone releasing hormone* (LHRH), and it was the first of several modern man-made hormone therapies that revolutionized prostate cancer care. Later, a similar drug called LHRH antagonist was developed. If neither the LHRH or LHRH antagonists work against the prostate cancer, drugs called anti-androgens can be tried. If those fail as well, then estrogen or ketoconazole may be tried.

LUTEINIZING HORMONE RELEASING HORMONE AGONISTS

Luteinizing hormone releasing hormone, or LHRH, is probably the most common form of hormone therapy given to men with advanced prostate cancer.

Also called LHRH agonists, this medication is given by injection in the doctor's office about once a month, or sometimes even less frequently.

Like estrogen, LHRH works by controlling the pituitary gland's release of luteinizing hormone, the hormone that spurs testosterone production in the testicles. The body's own natural LHRH is made in an area of the brain just next to the pituitary called the hypothalamus.

In healthy men, LHRH from the hypothalamus stimulates the pituitary gland to make LH. LH is released into the blood by the pituitary gland and stimulates the testes to make the hormone testosterone that is released into the blood. There is an ingenious check to the system: The testosterone in the blood causes the pituitary gland to temporarily stop making LH and that, in turn, temporarily turns off production of testosterone. When the blood level of testosterone drops again (after the testosterone is used up on its other tasks), then LH is released again and the process resumes. That happens about every 20 minutes in normal men.

When an LHRH agonist is given, for the first few days it acts alongside natural LHRH from the hypothalamus, causing an increased production of LH by the pituitary and parallel jump in testosterone production, known as a flare. During this time, some men may experience increased prostate cancer symptoms such as bone pain. (An anti-androgen may be prescribed before starting LHRH agonists to reduce this problem.) After the flare, the cells of the pituitary gland become exhausted from the continued bombardment of LHRH and they stop releasing LH. With no LH telling the testes to get busy, the production of testosterone in the testes stops.

These drugs are long-acting and can last from 1 to 6 months. Some men like the support of seeing the physician more often and want a monthly injection; others are inconvenienced by frequent doctor visits and prefer the longer-acting injection. LHRH drugs include Lupron epot and Trelstar. They can be given once every month, 3 months, or 4 months via an injection into the buttocks. Others are injected into the abdomen, such as Zoladex. It is important to realize that it takes 4 to 6 months after a LHRH therapy is stopped for testosterone levels to return to normal—maybe even longer in men older than age 70 years. This is both a pro and a con for LHRH agonists. It may take a while to be rid of the side effects of treatment if you stop, but it also means that a patient who is on LHRH agonists for many years can skip a treatment for a few weeks or months, and it should not make a difference to the growth of the cancer. The side effects of lack of testosterone production are the principal negatives related to chronic LHRH agonist treatment. (*See* pages 140–148 for a thorough review of ADT side effects and how to manage them.)

LHRH Antagonists

A second family of drugs, the LHRH *antagonists*, is now available again. (An earlier LHRH antagonist called Abarelix, product name Plenaxis, was withdrawn from the U.S. market in 2005 because of low sales). The new LHRH antagonist, Degarelix (product name Firmagon), was approved by the FDA in 2008 and so far has had a limited role in the hormonal treatment of prostate cancer. However, it is shaping up to be a popular option for ADT therapy. Like its predecessor, this LHRH antagonist directly blocks the effect of the natural

---

Agonist or Antagonist?

The names of two different forms of ADT are confusingly similar, LHRH agonists and LHRH antagonists, but they work in different ways. A drug that is an *agonist* is one that imitates the effect of a naturally occurring substance, such as a hormone, binding to the receptors on a cell just like the hormone to cause an effect. In this case, the LHRH agonist imitates the body's own luteinizing hormone, causing a lot of testosterone production until the whole production factory burns out. An *antagonist*, on the other hand, blocks the cell receptors, and prevents the naturally occurring hormone (or other substance) from doing its job. Therefore, an LHRH antagonist blocks the body's LHRH from connecting with other cells and passing on its message of testosterone production.

A Patient's Story: Hormone Therapy

Reggie M. was diagnosed with prostate cancer at age 59 years. He had skipped his physical only one year; when he went the next year, his PSA had jumped from 2 to 11. "You go through a cocktail of emotions," said Reggie about his diagnosis. "I had no symptoms; none whatsoever." After his prostatectomy, the pathologist found cancer cells in his seminal vesicles, so he was sent for postoperative radiation. Afterward, his PSA dropped and then started to rise again a year later. The scans showed nothing and his bone scans were clear. "The most stressful part was running those scans. Not invasive, but they scare the hell out of you." As his PSA crept up, ADT was his only option. Treatment, but not a cure. "There's no magic bullet, no chemo, that's what scares me," said Reggie, whose wife has had breast cancer twice and who watched his mother, his grandfather, and two other close relatives die of cancer. "It's the one death I did not want to undergo . . . I'd rather get hit by a car."

But today Reggie is very much alive. When he went on Lupron 5 years ago, his PSA went down instantaneously. A few years after that, his doctor added Casodex and Reggie remains healthy. He is surrounded by a supportive family, a trusting relationship with his doctor, and many friends and colleagues. "You count your blessings," he said. "It could be a lot worse."

LHRH released by the hypothalamus, which inhibits the release of LH from the pituitary gland. Without being told to manufacture testosterone via the LH from the pituitary gland, the testes don't manufacture anything. The result is the same decreased production of testosterone.

One selling point to these drugs is that they do not have an initial flare reaction because they block the release of LH from the pituitary without first causing an increase in the hormone, with its resultant increase in testosterone production. The ADT side effect profile will otherwise be the same as the LHRH agonist drugs because of the side effects caused by no testicular testosterone production.

Anti-Androgens

LHRH agonists and antagonists stop the testicles from producing testosterone, but a smaller amount of testosterone is also manufactured in the adrenal glands. That means even if a man is on LHRH therapy, there could still be some amount of testosterone floating around that is feeding the prostate cancer cells. Anti-androgens are a family of drugs that block entry of testosterone into the cells. This effectively starves any remaining prostate cancer cells of their testosterone fuel.

Anti-androgens have several roles in treating advanced prostate cancer. One use is to block the sudden flare of testosterone during the first few weeks after an LHRH agonist is given. The anti-androgens protect organs that may be infiltrated with prostate cancer cells, where even a small increase in the number of cancer cells would have a negative effect, like in the spinal cord or brain. Once the testosterone levels have dropped, it is not necessary to continue the anti-androgens as combined therapy with the LHRH agonist drugs—with one significant exception.

Because the anti-androgen drugs also block the effect of the 5% to 10% of circulating testosterone-like or androgen hormones that are produced in the adrenal glands, if the PSA levels do not go to undetectable levels over a few months of LHRH agonist therapy, then anti-androgen therapy should be added. The use of anti-androgens and LHRH therapy is known as complete androgen blockade (CAB) or maximum androgen blockade. Complete androgen blockade can be used if the LHRH drugs do not lower the testosterone levels sufficiently, or if the tumor continues to grow in the face of the ADT. Each of the anti-androgen drugs are taken as pills on a daily basis; some of the commonly prescribed anti-androgens are Cyproterone acetate, Flutemide, Nilutamide, and Bicalutamide.

Another possible use of the anti-androgens is to use the drugs alone as primary hormone therapy. That has been tried in some trials with reasonable success but is not done much yet in the real world. The dosage of anti-androgen used (bicalutamide) was 150 mg a day.[14] In small studies they have shown no difference in progression of disease between anti-androgen monotherapy and surgical castration. The incidence of loss of libido and hot flashes was lower, but the rate of painful breast growth greater, in the anti-androgen group.

One of the problems with the use of anti-androgens, and ADT in general, is cost. The suggested dose of Casodex (an anti-androgen) for hormone therapy is 150 mg/day. A month's supply of a 50-mg/day dose is $650, or about $32 per day. A 150-mg/day dosage would be impossible for most people if not covered by insurance. A 3-month supply of Lupron (a LHRH agonist) is $2900 (almost $1000 a month) and is covered by insurance in the United States. A generic version of Casodex, bicalutamide, is now available at a cost of $50 per month.

Another downside of anti-androgen use is a syndrome called the Anti-Androgen Withdrawal Syndrome. In 1993, there was a report that showed that some men receiving CAB, whose PSA continued to increase, experienced a drop of PSA for 5 months when the anti-androgen was stopped. It is not known why that happened. The clinical practice now is to stop anti-androgens if the disease is progressing, as measured by continuous rise of PSA. About a one-fourth of men have this reaction.

Ketoconazole

If the removal or switching of anti-androgens does not prove successful, or fails after a time, then the next thing to try is a drug called ketoconazole, which suppresses the production of the testosterone by the adrenal glands. Ketoconazole also suppresses production of testosterone by the testicles, but many experts advise continuing with LHRH agonist/antagonist treatment as well.

Ketoconazole, which has a trade name of Nizoral, is taken by mouth, and should be accompanied by a small dose of cortisone (a steroid) to replace the natural cortisone no longer produced by the adrenal glands. Ketoconazole is normally taken in a daily dose of 1200 mg divided into three parts and accompanied by a dose of 30 mg of cortisone. Incidentally, pharmacists frequently

balk at filling a prescription for such a large dose and often will require confir-
mation from the oncologist. Ketoconazole should ideally be taken with an
acidic type of food such as orange juice or tomatoes, which help the body absorb
the medication. It is also important for doctors to monitor the patient's liver
function, as ketoconazole can be toxic to the liver. It can also cause other strange
side effects such as anorexia and sticky skin.

The effectiveness of ketoconazole on the prostate cancer can last from a few
months to as long as 2 years, depending on the types of cancer cells present. If
problems such as liver toxicity occur with the high dosage mentioned above,
some success has been achieved with a reduced dosage of about one-half the
normal amount. This "low-dose keto" approach could be considered as an alternative. If that does not prevent the progression of PSA and cancer growth, some
chemotherapy might be given. Unfortunately, current chemotherapy is not very
effective on prostate cancer and extends life for advanced prostate cancer
patients only in months.

Making the Decision

There are no clear answers to the question of the timing and choice of hormone
therapy, either as LHRH agonist (or antagonist) drugs, anti-androgens on their
own, or combined anti-androgen–LHRH therapy, for men with advanced prostate cancer. On the pro side for making a quick decision to start ADT, there is
evidence to show a decrease in cancer progression and increase in overall survival with ADT—as well as reduction in the symptoms that are caused by the
disease such as difficulty urinating, urinary urgency, and frequency. On the con
side, there are the many side effects from ADT that clearly reduce the quality of
life. The choices are individual ones that should be made after discussion with
the caring physician and spouse and/or family or friends.

SIDE EFFECTS OF HORMONE THERAPY

Although ADT is the best line of defense for men with metastatic prostate
cancer, it may have serious, adverse effects on the quality of life. Testosterone is

---

CHEMOTHERAPY

Whereas ADT is based on the withdrawal of male hormone as a means of
killing cancer cells, chemotherapy relies on drugs that are very toxic–both

to cancer and to other rapidly growing cells. Chemotherapy is offered to men whose cancers have become *castration resistant,* that is those men whose prostate cancer seems to grow even in the presence of very low blood levels of testosterone. In the last 10 years the chemotherapy treatment most used for prostate cancer has been a drug called docetaxal, which is given in a series of 10 treatments, along with a steroid, prednisone.

Most urologists refer their patients who are castration resistant to medical oncologists. The oncologists specialize in giving chemotherapeutic agents to people with a wide range of cancers. At this time docetaxal provides a two- to three-month survival advantage over non-curative drugs. There are several new families of drugs on the horizon that are in late stage of testing or recently FDA-approved that may change the picture, including immune therapy.

Immune Therapy

On April 29, 2010 the Food and Drug Administration approved the first vaccine-like (immunologic) therapy for control of "hormone refractory" prostate cancer in men who have no or minor symptoms. (Hormone refractory cancer refers to cancer at a stage when the withdrawal of the testosterone no longer stops the growth of the cancer cells.) The therapy involves harvesting the patient's most active immune cells (called dendritic cells) and adding to them a specially-constructed protein that in turn will promote the body to generate an immune response to its own cancer cells.

The good news is that this technique has been shown to have some limited success in treating prostate cancer for men who have no other options. The bad news is that the treatment is expensive—$93,000 for one treatment—and the response is limited to about 4 months. An earlier trial in which the therapy was given to *symptomatic* men showed only a slightly greater improvement compared to placebo. Perhaps the most important aspect of this FDA approval is that it opens a door to other scientific pioneers who may now be able to obtain the funding needed to develop other improved immune treatments for cancer. Another form of promising therapy now in late stages of clinical testing is based on the idea that the castration-resistant prostate cancer cells have adapted themselves to function well even when the low blood testosterone levels should make them die. The new family of drugs, one of which is called Tokeda-100 (or TK-100), may further reduce the level of blood testosterone and disrupt the internal mechanism of the cancer cell so that it can no longer function. The importance of these new chemotherapy drugs to the man who has castration resistant prostate cancer is that positive advances are happening that will offer hope in the near future.

the hormone that gives men the feeling of maleness, including the desire to have sex (libido) and possibly the quality of erections; it also supports muscle mass and red blood cell and bone growth. Therefore, the decision to remove testosterone must be taken quite seriously, particularly because this treatment usually has to be used for the rest of the man's life to control the cancer. The principal side effects of removing testosterone from the blood include:

1. Loss of libido and sexual function (impotence)
2. Increased risk of cardiovascular disease
3. Increased risk of diabetes mellitus
4. Changes in body appearance: shrinkage of the testes, loss of body hair, enlargement of breast tissue
5. Decrease in bone density and a risk of osteoporosis
6. Decrease in muscle strength
7. Hot flashes
8. Weight gain
9. Anemia
10. Cholesterol and lipid increase

There are other possible side effects as well, including fatigue and general aches and pains. Research has shown that exercise programs can improve both muscle aches and lack of energy. Other possible symptoms from ADT treatment are still being studied, such as a decrease in memory and the ability to think, particularly in older patients (older than 75 years).[15] No research has focused on prostate cancer patients and memory loss specifically, so there is little data at this point, although some preliminary work seems to suggest that some types of memory might actually improve whereas others worsen.

Managing the Side Effects of Androgen Deprivation Therapy

Some men on hormone therapy begin to feel that they would have rather taken their chances with the cancer than endure the side effects of treatment. Let's face it: the side effects of ADT are not wonderful, but being alive is wonderful and ADT is what keeps men with advanced prostate cancer alive. To make that life more pleasant, you can address the side effects you experience with some of the treatment options below.

LOSS OF LIBIDO AND ERECTILE FUNCTION
Libido, the desire for sex, tends to be a hormone-dependent drive, and normal erectile function also depends on testosterone. The absence of testosterone

IMPORTANT MANAGEMENT STRATEGIES

Weight gain, body fat, triglycerides, and cholesterol are all increased in men on long-term LHRH agonist therapy.[i] Therefore, the risk of cardiovascular problems—particularly in older men on ADT—is of concern. The risk of serious cardiovascular problems, such as heart attack and stroke, occurs in one in five men on ADT and can begin in the first year after the treatment is begun.[ii] The rate of cardiovascular death in men on ADT was 5% as compared to 2% in men older than age 65 years who had had radical prostatectomy. This means that men on ADT must be aware of the potential problem and should make positive, proactive decisions to prevent further health problems.

A man can pursue a three-pronged strategy to help prevent or manage many, or even most, of his ADT side effects:

1. Maintain a healthy weight and protect existing muscle mass by eating a healthy diet high in protein, vegetables, grains and fruits, with moderate amounts of soy and flaxseed. (See page 159.)
2. Participate in a cancer support group—it is a free way to find out the inside scoop on how real men deal with these issues and can be very beneficial for your physical and mental health; you might find a workout buddy or learn a new way of thinking about your situation.
3. If you are not already doing so, institute a regular exercise regime that includes some weight-bearing exercises to preserve muscle mass and prevent osteoporosis and weight gain. I usually recommend at least 30 minutes of physical activity a day and weight lifting or resistance exercises (such as push-ups) several times per week.

If you can afford it, or if your insurance covers it, it could be very beneficial to meet with a nutritionist, a personal trainer, and maybe even a therapist during your hormone therapy to maximize your physical and mental well-being during this difficult time.

[i] Mohile SG, Mustian K, Bylow K, Hall W, & Dale W: Management of complications of androgen deprivation therapy in the older man. *Crit Rev.Oncol.Hematol.* 2009; 70: 235–255.

[ii] Saigal CS, et al. Androgen deprivation therapy increases cardiovascular morbidity in men with prostate cancer. Cancer. 2007;110:1493–1500.

tends to decrease libido in most men, so that some may not be as bothered about the accompanying sexual dysfunction. In some cases, the timing of this loss can coincide with a female partner's libido decrease after menopause, so that the couple is "in synch" sexually and more or less content with their less sexual relationship. In other cases, the spouse may want to be sexual, and her libido drives the man to seek help. A small number of men on ADT do continue to have libido and some erections; it depends on the degree of sexual drive present prior to treatment. Highly sexual men may be less affected by ADT than men with limited or reduced sexual drive.

If you are experiencing loss of libido, then one of the most effective ways to address the problem is through couples counseling with your partner or meetings with a sex therapist. You may not be able to return to your previous sex life, but there may be ways of preserving what you value in your intimate relationship (*see* Chapter 10 for practical tips). If you do maintain some libido, you may be able to return to erectile function by pursuing some of the treatments outlined in Chapter 4. Intracavernous injections and penile prostheses are two treatments that have a high level of effectiveness that does not depend on the presence of sexual desire.

One note: PDE-5 inhibitors like Viagra do not affect libido and are less effective in the presence of hormone suppression therapy. The action of the these drugs is to relax smooth muscle cells in the penis, and they tend to work better in the presence of some minimal erection—that is, they do not necessarily cause erection but will enhance and prolong it if the erection is initiated by other factors. Men with very high sex drive may still get (milder) erections. If they are still sexually active and start to get excited, then PDE-5 inhibitors will probably work. It is an individual process—there is no harm in trying it if you wish to have an erection, but don't think it will be a magic bullet.

> "It's not that [loss of libido and erections] doesn't bother me—but it is what it is. I'm happy to be alive."
>
> —Frank S.

CHANGES IN BODY APPEARANCE

Decreasing testosterone in the body can wreck havoc in many ways, both visible and invisible. To a man on ADT, the visible changes in his body may be among the most alarming side effects. The lack of testosterone can bring some more womanly features, such as an increase in the size of breast tissue. Brief radiation treatment of the breast area can sometimes forestall breast tissue enlargement. There are also some undergarments on the market that can minimize their appearance under clothing.

Shrinkage of the testicles occurs in almost every man undergoing ADT.

> "Not only did the hormone pills enlarge my breasts, but I even got a benign lump in one of them!"
>
> —Frank S.

The bulk of the testicles are tubules (basically groups of cells that hope to one day grow up to be sperm); the sperm-making cells in the tubules depend on testosterone for their growth. When ADT lowers testosterone supply, it shrinks these cells and the tubules. Sometimes the penis appears to decrease in size slightly as well. As discussed on page 123, this can sometimes occur after a prostatectomy alone. Unfortunately, there is not much that can be done about this side effect of ADT, except to adjust to the change while undergoing therapy. If you recover to a degree that you are able to discontinue ADT, then you mayeventually regain any size lost.

The loss or thinning of body hair on the arms and legs is also a common side effect of testosterone deprivation. Perhaps one of the oddest side effects of ADT is the reshaping of a man's pubic hair—from the male diamond to an inverted triangle shape similar to a woman's. Hair, or lack of it, may be a battle some men are willing to concede, or it may worry them intensely.

It is important to remember that depriving your body of testosterone does not turn you into a woman. You will continue to have male characteristics such as a lower voice, facial hair, and a fondness for the Three Stooges. In this regard, joining a support group of men also on hormone deprivation therapy can be very constructive. Talking with others who have fought the same battles you are facing can give you comfort, a feeling of camaraderie and of being understood, and good old-fashioned practical advice.

DECREASE IN BONE DENSITY AND AN INCREASED RISK OF OSTEOPOROSIS

Osteoporosis is the loss of bone density and actual bone mineral content. Men who have had surgical castration or who are using the LHRH agonist form of ADT are at risk for osteoporosis. The risk of bone fractures—particularly hip and spine—is a major health concern in an elderly population, because a major broken bone can lead to prolonged inactivity or bed rest, which in turn can lead to pneumonia or worse. For men on LHRH agonists, the risk of bone fracture is two to three times higher than in an age-matched group. Men on such therapy should have bone density tests done every several years. Men who follow the increased exercise and calcium regimen should not have that problem, but the longer the time on ADT, the greater the risk for osteoporosis and fracture.[16]

To help prevent osteoporosis, men on ADT are encouraged to quit tobacco and alcohol and increase their weight-bearing exercise to keep their bones strong. They should also consume a daily total of 1000 to 1500 mg of calcium and 400 to 800 IU of Vitamin D supplements, or calcium-rich, but low-fat foods (think Cherry Garcia® frozen yogurt instead of the full-fat ice cream version). If the bone density is found to be abnormally low, modern treatment includes injections of biphosphonate, a medication that can prevent and correct the problem.[17]

DECREASE IN MUSCLE STRENGTH

Testosterone in men is needed for muscle bulk. That is why professional athletes use testosterone-like steroid drugs to "bulk-up" and increase their athletic prowess. Testosterone actually increases the size of the skeletal muscle cells (muscles like your biceps or quadriceps, not muscles like your heart). Without testosterone, these muscles decrease in size and strength. It is therefore important that men on ADT try to increase their muscle strength with resistance exercise or weight lifting, if possible. (*See* the Appendix for exercise resources.) Some nutritionists also caution men (especially older ones) to keep an eye on their protein intake. Occasionally men in this situation experience a decrease in appetite, which often makes easier-to-digest carbohydrates seem more appealing. Eating plenty of lean protein, whole grains, and vegetables can help maintain your muscle tone and energy level.

HOT FLASHES

Hot flashes, or hot flushes, are one of the most frequent side effects of ADT that can have a significantly negative effect on quality of life. Hot flashes are sudden uncomfortable sensations of warmth or heat in the face, neck, upper chest, and back that may be accompanied by flushing or redness, sweating, nausea, and anxiety. In duration, they are characterized as lasting less than 1 minute, less than 5 minutes, or more than 5 minutes. No one actually knows the cause of hot flashes, although clearly they are related to a change in hormone levels that seem to have an effect on the hypothalamus, a part of the brain that regulates body heat. Not knowing the specific cause of hot flashes means that they are difficult to treat and the remedies that do exist are not very specific. Triggers that cause the hot flash may include heat, stress, change in body position, or drinking hot liquids.

The treatment is similar to those used to treat post-menopausal hot flashes in women. You should record the number, intensity, and length of the flashes and bring this record with you when you discuss treatment with the doctor prescribing your ADT. The recommended therapies begin with alternative or complementary ones that may help with mild or moderate flashes (infrequent flashes lasting less than 5 minutes). Those therapies include acupuncture and supplements, such as soy or crushed flaxseed. Black cohosh, a plant related to the buttercup, was also recommended at one time, but a recent National Institute of Health study showed it was not effective in post-menopausal women and recommended it be avoided.

Low-dose estrogens in the form of pills, patches, gels, creams, and injections may help hot flash symptoms. The other female hormone, progesterone, also seems to be of value as a low-dose pill, injection, patch, gel, or cream. Megesterol acetate and depot medroxyprogesterone acetate are female menstrual cycle hormones that have been used and reported to reduce the flashes by 85%.[18] The side effects of the progestational drugs can include weight gain, salt retention, and sexual dysfunction. Non-hormonal treatments have included the use of anti-depressants in the selective serotonin reuptake inhibitors (SSRI), anti-anxiety family of drugs, such as Paxil and Prozac, and a frequently used anti-convulsant drug, gabapentin, that is used for other medical problems such as anxiety and neuropathic pain. These are safe and worth a try, but there are few scientific studies to confirm their effectiveness in this case. (However, they may be an apt choice if you are also having anxiety.)

WEIGHT GAIN

Weight gain related to ADT may occur because low levels of testosterone are associated with the onset of the metabolic syndrome, a group of changes in the body that result in increase in body fat (particularly in the abdomen) and type II (adult-onset) diabetes. Increased exercise, weight lifting, resistance exercise, and dietary changes (particularly low-fat, low-carbohydrate diet) are strongly recommended for ADT patients to reduce their chance of heart attack and stroke.

ANEMIA

In men, testosterone affects red blood cell production in bone marrow. Too high a level of testosterone causes too high a red blood cell count, and too little testosterone can cause a low blood count known as anemia. Some studies estimate that as many as 90% of patients on ADT experience some level of anemia, usually a mild case that causes few problems. The anemia may begin about 6 months after starting therapy, and if the man exhibits anemia symptoms such as fatigue and breathlessness with minimal exercise, then treatment may be given. The subcutaneous injection of recombinant human erythropoietin, an available drug that can be given by the physician, seems to correct the problem.[19]

CHOLESTEROL AND LIPID INCREASE

ADT can often lead to an increase in low-density lipoprotein (LDL; or "bad") cholesterol levels. This, along with a higher risk of weight gain and type II diabetes, can place ADT patients at higher risks for cardiovascular "events" such as heart attack and stroke. The best first defense is to make any needed changes to a heart-friendly diet that is low in saturated fats and high in fiber.

Regular aerobic exercise (under a health professional's guidance) can also help. If your cholesterol levels do not respond, then statin medication such as Lipitor can be initiated to lower lipids. Any other outstanding heart issues, such as high blood pressure, should be carefully monitored and treated during hormone therapy. Make sure you have a risk assessment of lipids and blood pressure by your internist before treatment begins and that your oncologist or urologist is aware of any pre-existing heart conditions. In the presence of any heart issues, you should definitely check in periodically with your primary care physician or cardiologist while on ADT.

At the end of the day, hormone therapy is the only treatment proven to prolong life for advanced prostate cancer.[20] Whether you choose to accept ADT or not, when and what kind of ADT you choose is all up to you and your medical and support team. The important thing is to be at peace with your decision and live the best life you can. In Chapter 9, we will discuss the psychological impact of prostate cancer—strategies to deal with the stress of the situation and warning signs of the depression and anxiety that often accompany this disease.

Psychological Aspects of Prostate Cancer and Recovery

Whenever we experience a change in our physical health, it is natural to feel out of sorts emotionally, too. There are many reasons for this: being sick usually means an interruption in our normal lives—we don't have the comfort of our routine, our work, and regular social contact. It is common to feel at least a little helpless, because your body is doing things you don't want it to (feeling nauseated, growing cancer cells). You may have to visit uncomfortable places you really don't want to be (like doctors' offices and hospitals), where you have conversations you don't want to have about symptoms you don't enjoy having. If you have pain, fatigue, or other unpleasant symptoms, you are likely to feel down just from the physical sensations; you might want to withdraw from others until you feel "like yourself" again, until things go back to normal.

So what happens if there is an illness that doesn't go away so quickly? An illness like prostate cancer gives each patient a "new normal" to adjust to. For some lucky patients, the new normal is a temporary (weeks or months long) change, after which life pretty much goes back to its old rhythms. For others, it is a more long-term, more wrenching, change in lifestyle. It is perfectly normal to feel angry, scared, anxious, or depressed when dealing with cancer treatment and its aftermath. Added to that, there is stigma associated with prostate cancer—because it is seated in the genitalia, and because the side effects can involve bodily excretions and sex, which can make it more difficult to talk about, which in turn can lead men to hold it in and suffer in silence. They may think they are saving themselves more embarrassment. In actuality, most men who do take steps to improve their lives find that the embarrassment passes quickly and are surprised at how much things can improve in a short time.

Some prostate cancer patients simply accept the cancer, treatment, and treatment side effects as the price that must be paid to continue living.[1] But it is difficult to be so philosophical all the time. Most men will experience some distress associated with the cancer. The most common emotional reactions are anxiety and depression. These can be fleeting feelings, or they can develop into something that seriously impacts your daily life. Either way, they are treatable conditions, and you do not simply have to live with them. There are other common emotional states that can come up during this process; the important thing is to find ways to cope with them that work for you.

ANXIETY

A common accompaniment to a cancer diagnosis is a case of anxiety. Most men start having their PSA tested around age 50. Some men begin worrying about the results the minute their blood is drawn; others don't give it a second thought—until a high number comes back. For some men, a prostate cancer diagnosis is preceded by months or even years of annoying symptoms. Others have no symptoms at all and are blindsided by the diagnosis. No matter what your circumstances, the word "cancer" coming out of your doctor's mouth was probably a big shock. Cancer is a loaded word that can symbolize a loss of vitality and youth, independence, or even life. Even if you were able to focus on the promising statistics (although 30% of men older than age 50 years are diagnosed with prostate cancer, only 3% will die from the disease[2]) you probably still felt worried about how your cancer experience would play out.

Any kind of illness can cause worry, but prostate cancer has a few special quirks of its own that can throw patients for a loop. For one thing, there is no way for doctors to tell whether your tumor is very slow-growing and hence a good candidate for the "wait-and-see" approach or whether it is an aggressive cancer that could grow quickly and be much more life-threatening. Partly for this reason, men may feel pressured to make a quick decision about treatment. Depending on what kind of doctor you went to for follow-up, you may be nudged toward surgery (if you are seeing a urologist) or radiation (if you are seeing a radiation oncologist)—it is natural for specialists to believe most strongly in their own specialty, but it can leave you without all the information you would really like to have. With many contradictory and confusing statistics out there, it is not easy to compare treatment options on your own, which can add to your uncertainty and worry: Is this really the best option? What if it's not? Just when you've made peace with your treatment decisions, the aftermath of treatment often hits men where it hurts the most: even if you beat the cancer, you may have side effects of the most embarrassing kind. The uncertainty of not being able to rely on your body for the simplest things like continence and erections can be demoralizing.

Added to the physical uncertainty is a layer of social stigma that many men have a hard time breaking through. They may feel like they can't talk to anyone about the problems they're having because they're too embarrassing. They may even be reluctant to bring up erectile dysfunction or incontinence issues with their spouse—or even their doctor. Some men would rather "go it alone" than put their problems into words and pursue treatments to improve their condition. For that matter, some doctors (and other healthcare workers) are also embarrassed to bring it up and can tend to gloss over such topics quickly, or ignore them completely, rather than giving patients more opportunity to fully share what is going on. The silence that surrounds these side effects may have the effect of increasing anxiety because silence means less information, and less information (from doctor and patient) leads to decreased understanding. Decreased understanding might mean confusion . . . or believing some alarming "facts" about your condition that you read on the Internet that aren't really true. Silence can also add to feelings of being completely alone with your changed body, and that won't help your anxiety levels, either.

Finally, there is the worry of recurrence. For some prostate cancer patients, the disease becomes a long-term one. Every 3 months, they walk into their doctor's office to hear their new number. Will their PSA go up again? How much? It is very difficult to live under the strain of this anxiety, but many men do and live good lives in between those doctor visits.

To give an idea of how common it is to feel anxious in this situation, consider this: According to the National Institutes of Health, about one-third of prostate cancer patients suffer from serious anxiety[3]—that's about *10 times* more than similarly aged American men without cancer. You are not alone in feeling the way you do, and better yet, there are actions you can take that can help you feel less anxious.

DEPRESSION

Depression is the second most common mental health condition experienced by patients with cancer diagnoses, which often brings with it thoughts of mortality and decline. Depression can appear at any time during your cancer experience. Some patients feel most seriously down right after diagnosis. Others are distracted by all the treatment activity and the depression hits them after cancer treatment ("I've been *doing something* about this for the past few months—and now what?") For others, it can come and go without a pattern. Still others make it through treatment and post-treatment without much problem, only to be depressed by a recurrence.

Depression is characterized first by a persistent depressed mood (no energy, sad or tearful, loss of appetite). Of course, every cancer patient will have moments of feeling down, but when the feelings won't lift or are impairing your daily function (such as affecting your eating or sleeping habits), you may have crossed the line from a passing mood into depression. Note that depression is closely linked with pain.[4] Chronic pain can often cause depressed mood, and depression can trigger backaches and headaches that are otherwise unexplained. If you are in pain from your cancer or treatment, be vigilant for signs of depression.

Approximately *15%* of men with prostate cancer meet the criteria for clinical depression.[5] This is about 5 times the number found in the general population of older men in this country. Most urologists and oncologists do not monitor their patients for problems like depression and anxiety. (Indeed, studies have found that oncologists recognize depression in less than half of their depressed patients.)[6] It is up to you, the patient, to speak up when you think you might have such an issue and request a referral for mental health professional. You can also try some of the suggestions for self-help on pages 158–165.

OTHER EMOTIONAL REACTIONS

Betrayal

> *"A lot of doctors make it sound like you're getting your tonsils out, then afterwards you feel like you've been hit by a meteorite because you're not expecting anything."*
> —Leah C., Patient's Wife

Some men feel betrayed because something (like their own bodies) or someone (like their doctor) they used to trust "betrayed" them. Many men talk about being completely unprepared for the side effects that arise after treatment. Most of the time, this can be put down to the doctor–patient interaction before treatment (*see* Chapter 10 for more on the doctor–patient relationship).

A doctor may avoid having a properly detailed conversation before treatment because he/she feels uncomfortable discussing the embarrassing side effects such as incontinence or sexual dysfunction. Many doctors, like general oncologists who often deal with more dangerous cancers on a daily basis, will downplay the seriousness of prostate cancer and its aftermath for the simple reason that most prostate cancer patients will come out of treatment *alive*. Or they may be worried that by hearing about worst-case scenarios, their patients will be discouraged from pursuing suitably aggressive treatment. Another possibility is that the doctor has legitimately tried to go over the possible after-effects, but it is the patient who has either shut down the conversation or simply been too overwhelmed to take in the information.

THE ROLE OF AGE

Researchers think that that many people (doctors, patients, and family members included) downplay prostate cancer side effects because of common stereotypes about older men. Prostate cancer most affects men older than age 65 years and some people believe—wrongfully—that problems such as incontinence and ED are a "natural" part of aging. Adding to the insult of these assumptions is that around age 65 to 70 years, most men are facing retirement and the loss of professional meaning or identity in their lives.[i] They may also be experiencing the deaths of friends or family members—all of which adds to the likelihood of feeling depressed, helpless, or alone.[ii] All of these factors make it harder, but more important, for you to stand up for yourself and pursue effective treatments to improve your quality of life.

[i] Pirl WF & Mello J Psychological Complications of Prostate Cancer. *Oncology* (Williston Park). 2002;16 (11):1448–1153; discussion 1453–1454, 1457–1458, 1467
[ii] Kunkel EJ et al., Biopsychosocial Aspects of Prostate Cancer. *Psychosomatics* 2000;41(2), 85–94.

Either way, the result is the patient wakes up post-surgery, or a month after radiation, and realizes he has lost his urinary continence or erectile function, and he is angry. He may also feel betrayed because he hasn't been told about all the possibilities for rehabilitation of erectile and urinary function after treatment and may have lived through years of discouraging symptoms before finally finding help. Sometimes this will lead to a change of doctors or some uncomfortable moments during follow-up appointments. If you catch yourself acting out the anger on others around you, it is time to take steps for dealing with the anger in healthier ways. (*See* pages 158–169.)

Grief

When asked what one piece of advice she would give to prostate cancer patients and their partners, one wife of a patient replied, "Acknowledge the loss and never diminish it." Men, especially those who have never had a serious health problem before, will experience losses of many kinds. There is the loss of vitality and power over their own bodies that any illness brings. Prostate cancer and its treatments can bring other serious, sometimes permanent, losses: loss of an easy, spontaneous sex life; loss of continence; partial loss of masculine identity, confidence, sexuality; or maybe a loss of pleasure with your own body. Even small annoyances, when built up over time, can feel like loss; one patient wistfully remembered being able to wear khakis instead of dark pants only, as he does now that he has incontinence issues.

You don't want to wallow in your grief, as that can lead to depression, but you do want to pause and feel what you are feeling before pulling up on those bootstraps again. Pushing every sad moment under the mental carpet without addressing it can cause the grief to come out in less healthy ways, like irritation with family members, too much drinking, or even new physical health problems. There are many resources out there for people dealing with grief (*see* Appendix for possible resources). Don't fool yourself into thinking that there is nothing to be sad about—and don't get stuck in the sadness. Some sessions with a sympathetic ear of a counselor, or just sharing your feelings with a trusted friend, may relieve your pain (as might some of the treatment suggestions later in this chapter).

Guilt

Patients can feel guilty for various reasons during their cancer experiences. They may feel they should have done something to prevent the cancer in the first place—like get more regular check-ups or quit smoking. Or they may feel guilty that they chose a particular treatment without consulting their spouse or getting a second opinion. Most heartbreaking is when a patient feels guilty because of how his disease or treatment is affecting his relationship with another person. Many men are used to being the strong ones in a partnership and supporting their significant others through hard times. When such a man has to rely on support or even ask for help, he may feel guilty and out of sorts. In cases like this, being able to tell your spouse how you are feeling may be all you need to do to break through. In other cases, counseling alone or with your partner might help you come to terms with the new, perhaps temporary, change in your couples dynamic. In the next chapter, we will address the ways a relationship can change and strategies for staying close after prostate cancer.

Remorse

Remorse can hit when you begin to have second thoughts about the choices you made during your cancer experience. Perhaps you feel a different treatment would have been a better choice or perhaps you wish you had never pursued active treatment at all, but rather just waited to see if the tumor grew. As mother always said, it's easy to have 20/20 hindsight and "know" what the right decision was, looking back on it. It is harder to learn to live with the decisions you made, here in the present, instead of second-guessing the past. A shift in viewpoint is often useful: talking about your experience with a friend and hearing how he or

Table 9.1. RISK FACTORS

Some people are more likely to develop mental illness that requires treatment. The factors listed below can put men at a higher risk for depression or anxiety at this time. If you or a loved one falls into any of these categories, be especially vigilant for signs of distress.

- *Hormone therapy:* Men receiving hormone therapy are more likely to experience more mental and emotional stress.[a]
- *History of mental illness:* If you have had similar problems before, you know how useful treatment can be. If you have a history of untreated mental illness, cancer can be both a curse (in that it may cause a relapse) and a blessing (in that it gives you a chance to be healthier all around and choose to get help for all your medical issues).
- *History of trauma or recent losses:* New traumas associated with the cancer experience can trigger post-traumatic stress disorder or other psychological problems.[b] Prostate cancer and the losses associated with it may also compound recent losses to push simple sadness into real depression.
- *Social isolation, or poor support networks:* Going it alone may seem heroic at first but puts men at an increased risk for depression and other problems. Low social support is also associated with increased mortality.[b]
- *Poorly controlled pain:* As noted above, pain and depression are highly correlated. Researchers have found that 55% of prostate cancer patients report pain.[b]
- *Alcohol and substance abuse:* If you already use alcohol or drugs to "self-medicate" your emotional states, then cancer may really throw you into dangerous territory—mixing alcohol and treatment drugs, leading you deeper into depression, anger, or anxiety. You might find cancer also offers you an opportunity to make healthier choices all around.

[a] Bloch S et al., Psychological adjustment of men with prostate cancer: a review of the literature. *BioPsychoSocial Medicine* 2007; 1:2
[b] Kunkel EJ et al. Biopsychosocial Aspects of Prostate Cancer. *Psychosomatics* 2000; 41(2): 85–94.

> "I took the opportunity to stop drinking, so the date of my surgery is my sobriety anniversary, too. My first AA sponsor was also a prostate cancer survivor—which helped me, too."
>
> —Jake T.

she sees it could help you gain some perspective, as could talking with a counselor or distracting yourself with new productive activities in your life.

TREATMENTS

There is so much you can do to feel better; it is difficult to justify the route of doing nothing and continuing to feel bad. Some remedies are home remedies like your mother might have recommended; others are scientifically proven to be effective. In addition to a long list of easy-to-do actions, there are also a host of mental health professionals available to consult with and advise you on your journey back to yourself. If you feel hesitant about these first steps, consider this: As a patient, you wouldn't hesitate to tell your doctor a physical side effect you are having; your quality of life should be just as important to you. Also take strength in knowing how much your loved ones want you to be as happy as possible. If you can't do it for yourself, do it for them.

SELF-TREATMENTS

Depending on the severity of your symptoms, you might find considerable relief by taking some simple actions on your own. The actions listed below require no fancy equipment or expertise. Even patients with no mental illness at all can benefit from this advice, culled from patients, mental health professionals, and published psychological studies. For other men, especially those with the risk factors discussed above in Table 9.1, these actions may not be enough—or may not feel feasible—and a consultation with a mental health professional could offer better solutions.

Educate Yourself

Knowledge really is power. When you receive a cancer diagnosis, you are stepping into a strange new world, full of disorienting experiences, little paper robes, and big words that no one takes the time to explain. Feeling like you're not sure what's going on may add to a general feeling of helplessness that many patients have. These feelings are related to increased anxiety and depression.[7] To offset such feelings, arm yourself with information! Even if you're not a naturally upbeat person, educating yourself can help: studies have shown that information can help even normally pessimistic people feel better about their situation.[8]

Beware of the challenges to educating yourself, however, as you move forward. Every specialist believes most strongly in his own specialty. If you see a surgeon first, if your medical condition and age are appropriate, he or she is usually going to recommend you get surgery. Make sure you get more than one opinion before deciding on an irreversible course of action (they can't put that prostate back in). The information on the Internet about prostate cancer and side effects can be contradictory and confusing. Be very careful about which sites you trust. (You can find some good ones in the Appendix.) Sometimes your fellow patients are a great source of information. They can tell you what your doctors can't: How does it feel to have radiation every day for a month? Which brand of incontinence pads work best? How did they negotiate restarting intimacy with their partner?

Develop your Support Network

The top recommendation of most former prostate cancer patients is to bring a friend or family member with you to all your important appointments. When considering a new diagnosis or a course of treatment, four ears are better than two. Your spouse or friend may be less inhibited in asking questions or have medical knowledge that you don't.

If you don't feel close to your family, or don't live close to them, you'll need to build your own web

> "I didn't want this secret. I did at the beginning, but not anymore. I was embarrassed but it's hard to keep this kind of thing secret. People want to know how you are, what's going on . . . so you just face it. Look, everybody's got some sort of shit going on. Breast cancer, whatever, everybody's been touched by it. Like that story about the man who was complaining about his shoes until he met a man with no feet."
>
> —Jake T.

of support. Many patients start off thinking they are strong, independent souls who can handle it all on their own. At some point during treatment, aftermath, or recurrence, almost all have a change of heart and realize that there is simply a human need for other people, especially in times of trouble, no matter how strong and independent you are. Dozens of scientific studies have proven that married people have significantly better health outcomes than single people. This doesn't mean that if you're single, you're doomed; it means that you aren't married to your key support person and will have to make an effort to enlist friends or family members to provide a support net.

> *"I didn't talk to anybody for 2 years until I realized, 'What am I doing?' Hey, nobody talks about this stuff! So I started volunteering to talk to newly diagnosed patients."*
> —Richard D.

Talk About It

If you share your feelings with your cancer doctor, he or she may be able to adjust medication (especially if you are on hormone therapy) to lessen feelings of depression or anxiety. Your emotional state could also be a sign to them that a selected course of therapy needs some modifications to better serve your needs.

OR WRITE ABOUT IT

Some hospitals run writing groups for patients, as part of a national movement called "narrative medicine." I help facilitate such a group on the oncology ward at a hospital in New York. Because we focus on the craft of writing, we are not talking about feelings just to talk about feelings—we are there to create something constructive out of a disease that often feels destructive. We're definitely supportive, but it's not a support group. The participants in these workshops often feel empowered by narrating their own stories using their own words (not the doctors') and their own voices. Even just writing on your own, at home, can help you process your emotions and feel more in control. Other artistic pursuits such as painting and music might also feel especially meaningful right now. You might find yourself creating a work of art out of your cancer and recovery experience, turning loss into something beautiful.—Rosemary

Talking about your cancer, or your depression/anxiety, with friends and family may be surprisingly helpful—you may find that some of them have had the same feelings. This can be especially helpful when they have been through a bout of cancer or other serious illness.

Get Relief for Pain and other Symptoms

Untreated pain can severely impair your quality of life. Patients may feel like they don't want to complain or should "tough it out," but actually pain alone can cause people to isolate themselves and feel depressed. Don't count on your doctors to ask or notice (doctors typically underestimate the amount of pain their patients have); call them up, or bring it up at your next appointment, and keep bringing it up until you feel better. Similarly, fatigue often goes unnoticed by doctors and under-reported by patients. It can also lead to feeling "out of it" mentally, even without other medical problems. Again, talk to your doctor about medical solutions (adjusting your treatment schedule, or sleep medication) and take care of yourself by getting as much sleep as you need to feel better, without judging yourself as lazy or weak.

Re-Organize your Schedule as Needed

As much as possible, keep up with regular activities. Don't isolate yourself from your social and professional circles that can offer you structure and solace right now. However, if your regular schedule includes a lot of stress, try to reprioritize your time to make time for activities that make you feel better instead of worse.

Get Physical Exercise

There is much research that proves the value of exercise to mental health as well as physical. Not only do those cute little endorphin hormones make you feel

---

PROSTATE CANCER AND DIET

During your cancer treatment, it might feel like your medical team is literally calling the shots, while you sit on the sidelines. It is natural to want to *do* something to improve your own chances for a successful recovery, and many men turn to diet as an area of their life that they can use to favorably affect their prostate health.

There is clearly one thing you can do to benefit the health of your prostate and every other part of your body: *lose weight if you are overweight*. Obese men have a 54% higher chance of developing fatal or metastatic prostate cancer, compared to men of normal weight.[i] Other studies showed that while obese men were no more likely to get prostate cancer, they were more likely to die of it.[ii]

And healthier doesn't have to mean less yummy: research has shown that lycopene, a naturally occurring substance found in tomato sauce, watermelon, and papaya, seems to lower the risk of developing prostate cancer.[iii] Though not every study has confirmed this relationship, there is enough evidence to give you an excuse to layer the marinara sauce on your wholegrain pasta. To wash that down, reach for some green tea—data from European studies (not yet duplicated in the US) seems to support its benefits.[iv] A sprinkling of flaxseed on your morning cereal (or in your pancakes) and a glass of pomegranate juice may be prostate-healthy additions to your diet, too.[v],[vi]

When it comes to supplements, be a smart shopper. Some that were once touted as helpful (such as Vitamin D) have not had their benefits supported by research. Previous claims for selenium and vitamin E have not been supported–newer studies by the National Cancer Institute showed that neither had any power to reduce the risk of prostate cancer—in fact, it pointed to a possible increased risk of prostate cancer for men who took large doses of Vitamin E.[vii] Zinc was also once thought to be helpful but most recently has been associated with a *higher* risk of prostate cancer.[viii] The safest route is to save your money, keep within the daily-recommended range with vitamins and use caution with herbal supplements until the research is definitive.

In the meantime, lose any extra pounds, and eat sensibly: if you like tomato sauce and green tea then eat them. If you don't like them, don't feel you have to choke them down. By taking control of your weight and eating healthy foods that appeal to you, you have a good chance of positively impacting your prostate cancer recovery—and feeling better physically and mentally.

[i] Rodriguez C, Freedland SJ, Deka A, Jacobs EJ, McCullough ML, Patel AV, et al. Body Mass Index, Weight Change, and Risk of Prostate Cancer in the Cancer Prevention Study II Nutrition Cohort. Cancer Epidemiol. Biomarkers Prev. 2007: 16: 63–9.

[ii] Wright ME, Chang SC, Schatzkin A, Albanes D, Kipnis V, Mouw T, et al. Prospective study of adiposity and weight change in relation to prostate cancer incidence and mortality. Cancer 2007; 109: 675–84.

[iii] Giovannucci E, Ascherio A, Rimm EB, Stampfer MJ, Colditz GA, Willett WC. Intake of carotenoids and retinol in relation to risk of prostate cancer. J. Natl. Cancer Inst. 1995; 87: 1767–76. Key TJ, Appleby PN, Allen NE, Travis RC, Roddam AW, Jenab M, et al. Plasma carotenoids, retinol, and tocopherols and the risk of prostate cancer in the European Prospective Investigation into Cancer and Nutrition study. Am. J. Clin. Nutr. 2007; 86: 672–81.

[iv] Kurahashi N, Sasazuki S, Iwasaki M, Inoue M, Tsugane S; JPHC Study Group. Green tea consumption and prostate cancer risk in Japanese men: a prospective study. Am. J. Epidemiol. 2008; 167: 71–7.
Bettuzzi S, Brausi M, Rizzi F, Castagnetti G, Peracchia G, Corti A. Chemoprevention of Human Prostate Cancer by Oral Administration of Green Tea Catechins in Volunteers with High-Grade Prostate Intraepithelial Neoplasia: A Preliminary Report from a One-Year Proof-of-Principle Study. Cancer Res. 2006; 66: 1234–40.

[v] Demark-Wahnefried W, Polascik TJ, George SL, Switzer BR, Madden JF, Ruffin MT, et al. Flaxseed Supplementation (Not Dietary Fat Restriction) Reduces Prostate Cancer Proliferation Rates in Men Presurgery. Cancer Epidemiol. Biomarkers Prev. 2008; 17: 3577–87.

[vi] Pantuck AJ, Leppert JT, Zomorodian N, Aronson W, Hong J, Barnard RJ, et al. Phase II study of pomegranate juice for men with rising prostate-specific antigen following surgery or radiation for prostate cancer. Clin Cancer Res. 2006; 12: 4018–4026.

[vii] Gann PH. Randomized trials of antioxidant supplementation for cancer prevention: first bias, now chance–next, cause. JAMA 2009; 301(1): 102–3.

[viii] Leitzmann MF, Stampfer MJ, Wu K, Colditz GA, Willett WC, Giovannucci EL. Zinc supplement use and risk of prostate cancer. J. Natl. Cancer Inst. 2003; 95(13): 1004–7.

better, exercise can also prove that your body is still under your control—and remind you that you're not dead yet! Of course, you will probably not be up for marathons or long-distance bike rides, but with your doctor's okay, swimming, walking, racquetball, and other exercises can be very beneficial. Also exercises that have specific stress management components, such as yoga (it's tougher than you think), martial arts, or tai chi, can have a double impact on your mental outlook.

Consider Meditation, Prayer, or other Spiritual Practice

Any type of stress relief or "centering" practice can improve your mental outlook. All the better if you can tap into a spiritual place at the same time; many people find that regular prayer grounds them and helps them feel connected to something bigger than themselves. For those who aren't into the praying thing, there are plenty of non-faith-related routes to go for a similar positive effect. Even clearing a quiet space and time for 10 minutes a day when you sit and think of nothing (or do some visualization exercises) can bring great benefits to your mental and physical health. Simple instructions on beginning meditation can be found on the Internet or in how-to books.

DEVELOPING NEW INTERESTS

A serious illness can act like a "restart" button for your life. Always wanted to learn Italian or go parachuting? Why not do it now? Giving yourself license to try something new can give you a feeling of freedom and joy that might come in handy right about now. Frank S. retired about six months after his prostatectomy. "I took up new things: bought a boat, took up scuba diving, started traveling. When I started all these new activities, I almost forgot about [my prostate cancer problems]—I'd get so preoccupied with Mexico; it had me smiling, had me laughing. It felt good."

Set Realistic Goals

One of the complaints heard often from prostate cancer patients is that they are not prepared for what comes after the treatment. Sometimes doctors gloss over embarrassing topics like incontinence or ED. Sometimes patients are too overwhelmed by their situation to take in what their doctors are saying (another good reason to bring your spouse or a friend with you to your appointments). If you realize now that your ideas about your post-cancer life (e.g. to resume your pre-cancer sex life within a month of surgery) were not realistic, then there's no time like the present to take stock and make new goals. Re-adjust your ideas of what's possible for you *now*, in this new reality. With your partner, if you have one, explore different ideas about sex, such as focusing more on pleasure than performing a perfect 10. Talk with your doctor or mental health professional about what new goals you can set yourself that you can achieve in the near future. Reaching your goals, even if they are not your "ultimate" goal, will do a lot to help you feel more in charge, maybe more like your old self.

DO EVERYTHING YOU CAN TO DEVELOP A POSITIVE ATTITUDE

When asking prostate cancer patients what advice they had for current or new patients, a common refrain rose up. "Please emphasize one thing: It's having a positive attitude. Your mind has a lot of effect over how your body works. Keep focused on the positive parts of life." (Reggie M.) "Attitude is very important." (Michael K.) "Sometimes I'm approached by kvetchers and I ask them 'What good are you doing by only focusing on your problems?' I have the same remorse as anyone else has, but it's short-lived. I don't have the time for it." (Richard D.) Even if a positive outlook doesn't ultimately improve your outcome, you (and the people around you) will enjoy your life more now.

Join a Support Group—In Person or Online

Some men think support groups are crybaby parties for sissies and losers who can't "take it like a man." In reality, they are full of people like you—formerly healthy men who have been shocked by their diagnoses; men who are trying to deal with weird new side effects; men who are frustrated by their condition; men who are looking for information, understanding, or camaraderie.

It might not be easy the first time. Many people describe walking into the meeting room the first time as one of the hardest things they've ever done. But it can also be one of the best things you can do for yourself (and sometimes your partner—partners of PCA patients have formed their own groups in many regions). Of course, not everyone feels the need for support beyond their own family and friends, but support group friends can offer you something your wife or partner can't: they have had their prostates out, or had seeds put in, and lived through the aftermath. Support groups typically meet in hospitals or community centers and are led by a social worker or trained counselor who is very familiar with the issues specific to your disease. See the Appendix for more information on how to find a group in your area. Encourage your wife or partner to consider joining a group for loved ones of prostate cancer survivors.

The Internet can also offer some great opportunities to connect with men who have faced the same challenges. Blogs, chat rooms, and list serves can bring information and encouragement to your home computer. The Appendix lists some popular and useful websites that can get you started.

In addition to the emotional and informational benefits of joining a support group, several studies suggest that being part of a support group can improve your physical health "outcome"—that is, you may actually end up healthier all around, and living longer, because you chose to walk in that room for the first time.

> *"Support groups were so important for me. I did not want to go to them at first. But later, in that room with all these people, was like security or something. Plus I got so much information. I knew nothing at the beginning."*
>
> *—Frank S.*

An Important Note on Avoidance

Although it may be tempting to just ignore what's going on in your body (and your head), think twice before choosing this route. Psychological studies of cancer patients have proven that "avoidance of these issues [anxiety or depression] leads to increased suffering, significant psychological distress and feelings of despair, isolation, hopelessness, and passive thoughts of wanting to die."[9] Active attempts to "process" feelings and develop coping skills have been shown to be better for adjustment than denial.[10] Others found that social support, self-esteem, and feelings of empowerment all made a positive contribution to the prostate cancer adjustment process, whereas suppression of anger and depression did not.[11]

WHEN TO SEE A PROFESSIONAL

If you have tried some of the strategies above and nothing seems to work for you, you might consider a referral to a mental health provider. Obviously if you think you might hurt yourself or someone else, you should seek treatment immediately, preferably by calling 911. But you don't have to be at that point to benefit from a mental health consult.

How do you know if it is time to reach out for help? Basically, if your mental state is adversely affecting how you live your life, it is time to get treatment.

For example, is your anxiety over your PSA keeping you from making that follow-up appointment or giving you gut-wrenching stomachaches? Is your depression affecting your appetite or your sleep? Are activities that used to be fun no longer fun? Other signs that it is time to pick up the phone and make the therapy appointment: work absenteeism because of your mental state; social withdrawal; a new tendency to pick fights with family members or co-workers; increased use of alcohol or substance use.

The people around you may be trying to talk to you about some of these things—perhaps you are aware that your wife is pestering you more about your drinking or your boss is getting on your case about your attitude at work. Instead of tuning them out, take it as a sign that you need to consider changing your approach. The most important signal of all is one that only you are aware of: Are you upset by the way you are feeling? Do you wish you could get help? Well, here's good news—there is a lot of help available.

Mental Health Services

These days, the stigma of going to a mental health professional is almost non-existent. . . or at least it should be. A lot depends on where you live, your cultural background, and your own preconceptions about what psychologists or psychiatrists do. They will not try to brainwash you; rather, as one psychiatrist put it: "Our job is to get people back to themselves—what they see as themselves—and functioning at their best."

With the advent of more psychiatric drugs, plentiful advertising and consumer education has driven home the idea that mental illness is just that: an illness. It is not a sign of weakness (or "craziness") to consult a specialist about a health problem; it is smart. It is also more affordable than it ever was before. Recent federal and state laws are bringing our country closer to mental health insurance benefits that will match those for other medical problems.

Mental health professionals can also be partners in your physical care. For example, a psychologist could help you reframe sexual issues to improve your sex life or come up with coping skills to deal with UI. Although you may not want to add another medicine to your regime, psychiatric drugs could offer you additional physical benefits. For example, certain anti-depressants in low doses also help alleviate hot flashes suffered by men on hormone therapy.

Mental health treatment can last several sessions or several years, depending on your condition and the treatment approach. There may be less choice in rural areas than in cities, but there is almost always a community health option that provides low cost or sliding scale services. Personal recommendations from friends, family, or support group members can be helpful in finding a good practitioner. Don't be afraid to "shop around" if you don't click with the first doctor you go to. Just like any relationship, the strength of the doctor–patient rapport depends partly on chemistry. There are a variety of professionals that offer mental health services:

- *Psychiatrists:* Psychiatrists are MDs who have completed medical school like any other physician, and then do another 4 years of psychiatric training. They may have connections to hospitals or other medical facilities and can prescribe medications. Various specialties exist within the field, including psychopharmacology (psychiatric drugs), geriatric psychiatry, and addiction psychiatry. (Many men "self-medicate" for depression or anxiety using alcohol or other substances. If you think you might be doing this, see a professional as soon as possible before your problems multiply.) You might meet with a psychiatrist every week, or see her every month or so for a prescriptions, while seeing a psychologist or therapist for weekly sessions. ("Therapist" is a broad term that could mean a psychologist, counselor, or social worker.) If you prefer, or if there are no psychiatrists in your area, primary care physicians can also prescribe anti-depressants and other medications and help you find a good therapist.
- *Psychologists:* Psychologists typically have doctorates in psychology and are required to complete a lengthy training and licensing process before they can practice. Generally they cannot prescribe medication (but they are permitted to do so in New Mexico and Louisiana). Psychologists can offer tests, such as ones that can help pinpoint when a problem is a mental illness or a neurological one (e.g., dementia). They may focus on a particular type of psychotherapy, such as psychoanalysis (an intensive, introspective therapy that usually requires years of meeting several times a week). More commonly, psychologists have a more laid back approach than that, and a typical treatment would be to meet every week for an hour over the course of a few months.
- *Counselors:* "Counselor" is a broadly defined category, but anyone who does psychological counseling should have at least a master's degree in a relevant field (social work or psychology) and should have gone through a supervised training process to obtain a license to practice. Often counselors can be more affordable and every bit as good as a psychologist or psychiatrist, but be sure to inquire about the person's background before committing to a course of treatment. Like psychologists, a counselor would probably want to see you every week

for an hour-long session (many therapists have evening hours available as well).

- *Social workers:* Social workers can be a wonderful resource for any patient, because they can often help coordinate medical care or family issues in a very practical way. For example, they can connect you with local resources that might help you get transportation to appointments or find care for a child or an ill family member. Social workers usually have an master's degree in Social Work as well as practical experience. Sometimes they work in hospitals, specializing in helping a certain population (e.g., cancer patients); other times they work independently, more as a counselor than a hands-on problem solver.
- *Clergy:* Some people feel more comfortable confiding in a trusted clergy member of their own faith. Clergy may be certified as "pastoral counselors" who have training in mental health therapies (such as individual, family, or couples) in addition to their religious training. Often clergy are especially comforting to talk to as they can integrate faith-based solutions like prayer into treatment. They may also be well-connected in the community and able to offer practical assistance through the church or other local organizations.
- *Cognitive behavioral therapists:* Cognitive behavioral therapy (CBT) is usually a short-term therapeutic approach that focuses on behavioral change instead of more introspective exploration. That is, instead of focusing on feelings, CBT focuses on behavior and how we can get out of unhealthy behavioral habits. For example, in CBT you and your therapist might work out strategies to lessen the anxiety around follow-up appointments. Stress reduction and goal setting are often cornerstones of this approach. CBT can be very empowering for patients, whether they have an actual mental illness or just need some help getting through a particular experience, such as cancer treatment.
- *Couples therapists:* As the name suggests, couples therapy is about working out issues that arise in a marriage or romantic relationship. Usually couples therapy involves both partners going to the therapist together; sometimes the counselor might see them separately as well. This can be especially useful for prostate cancer patients and their partners who are trying to adjust to a new relationship dynamic or a new sex life (or lack thereof) that has been imposed by the illness. If you as a patient don't feel supported by your partner, or feel that there are communication difficulties in your marriage, then couples therapy could prove very useful. Most couples therapists will have either a master's or doctorate degree; many states require licensing, but some do not.

- *Sex therapists:* Sex therapy can be very useful for prostate cancer patients, whether or not they have a partner. This cancer strikes men at the very heart of their sexuality and can mean a dramatic shift in their identity as men and sexual beings. A sex therapist can help you (and your partner) come to terms with a new sexual normal and discover ways to still enjoy sex—even if it's not the exact same way you used to enjoy it. Such therapy is usually short-term. Sex therapists should have a master's or doctorate degree, as well as special training in sexual issues.

Developing new goals to improve your quality of life can take courage. Sometimes it is easier to take the first steps with your spouse, or a supportive friend, at your side. Whether or not you have a partner or spouse in your life, it is important to recognize that your mental state affects not just you, but those around you as well, and, potentially, your medical outcome. In the next chapter, we will look at how prostate cancer and its aftermath can impact key relationships in your life.

Prostate Cancer Recovery and Relationships

Your cancer experience is unique: no one will ever walk the exact same path as you will through your illness, your treatment, and the aftermath. Your cancer experience is not solitary, although it is true that only your blood gets drawn for the prostate-specific antigen (PSA) test and only your body that is attacked by the cancer cells. But it is not just your life that is changed. Your loved ones will suffer beside you, whether you want them to or not, because that's what we do when people we care about are going through a hard time.

Some of the worst possible outcomes from prostate cancer are broken marriages and cooled friendships. Your actions and attitude can affect what kinds of changes happen in your relationships during and after your prostate cancer treatment. There is a lot of stigma attached to this disease, which can lead many men to staying silent, even with their partners and closest friends. You may think you are saving your friends from worrying about you, but keeping quiet can also lead to misunderstandings that push people away. Friends may read your silence as a rejection of their concern—a big "Keep Out" sign on your feelings. Your wife may be thinking you have lost all interest in her but can't bring herself to ask. Keeping your relationships strong is under your control: your friends and family will take your lead on how to deal with you during this time. Good communication habits can help them understand your needs and desires and create a support network that can endure long beyond your cancer treatment.

Maintaining a strong support team means reaching out and opening up a little to your friends and family. This can be very difficult for many men. Below we offer a few strategies for talking about your cancer experience with the important people in your life in a way that is appropriate for the level of intimacy in the relationship. Later in this chapter, we will examine the changes that can happen between spouses and ways to keep your marriage or partnership strong.

FRIENDS, EXTENDED FAMILY, AND CO-WORKERS

It is both an advantage and a disadvantage that prostate cancer is easy to conceal from just about everyone. Most of the symptoms and treatment side effects are, by their nature, private. (Most people don't talk about erectile dysfunction on the bus.) Yet these same issues can weigh heavily on a person's psyche. If you do not have a life partner (and even if you do), think about choosing a few friends to confide in so that the weight of your illness can be shared and you have other people you can depend on for support when you need it. You may want help researching doctors, someone to pick you up after a radiation appointment, or just someone to go out to dinner with to take your mind off things.

Who to Tell and How

These questions are not easy to answer, and will vary for every man, but there are a few basic strategies to consider. First, you will want to share different things with different people. For example, you may tell your boss and co-workers a brief, honest explanation so they will understand any absenteeism. Then some friends, who aren't your closest, may get a little more information, but not full disclosure. But you are probably going to need one or two friends that you can *really* talk with. Your closest friends or family members—maybe a sibling or a best friend—would be a natural choice (Who was best man at your wedding? Who do you call when you have good or bad news to share?) There are some other points to take into account as well.

1. *Comfort with illness/body issues:* If your best friend can't even visit his sick mother in a hospital, then think twice about making him your main confidante. If he squirms at the mention of cancer, then you might look for someone else—perhaps another friend has been

through cancer or has helped a spouse weather it. A person who has spent time in hospitals and doctor's offices, either as a patient or caretaker, might better relate to your experiences. On the other hand, if the person is currently caretaking, then he or she might not have much energy left to give.

2. *Broad shoulders:* If you have the choice between someone who tends to be easily stressed out by life and someone who tends to be calm and steady: choose the person less likely to fall apart, either from worry about you or fear of the general situation.

3. *Attitude:* Some of us have sunnier outlooks than others. We all have at least one friend for whom the world is a dark, gloomy place. (Hint: That's not the person to ask for support right now.)

4. *Skills to match your needs:* Maybe what you need most is help understanding the medical lingo—in that case, you might talk to your brother-in-law who is a lab tech at a hospital. If you need someone with whom you can talk candidly about your marriage and sex life, consider a friend far away who is not likely to run into your wife (there's nothing that says your support can't come over the phone).

> "I got so much information from my friend Mike, who had been through it himself, but frankly, he was a bit of a downer. I would've preferred a cheerleader."
>
> —Jake T.

Some Tips for Cancer Conversations

Finding the words to start that first conversation can be difficult. If you are unsure of what kind of reception you will get, try to do it in person if possible, and pay attention to your friend's reaction: Does he show a lot of discomfort or listen attentively? Choose a good time and place. The 5 minutes before the coin toss in the football stadium might not be the best choice. You want to be somewhere where you can have a private conversation without worrying about being overheard and have enough time that you aren't looking at your watch while you talk.

FOR YOUR BOSS/CO-WORKERS

Unless you are very close, it might be best to have this conversation once you have decided on your treatment. That way you will have an excuse to bring it up, which is scheduling.

Sample opener: "You might have noticed I was out for some doctor's appointment last month. Well, I've just learned I have prostate cancer. It's not life-threatening and unlikely to affect my job. However, I will have to be out of the office when I go in for surgery—I'll need about a week or 10 days' time off for surgery and recovery."

> *"I was afraid for him and very protective of him. I wasn't sure we should tell anyone, but the flip side is: people are really nice when you need them."*
> —Leah C., Patient's Wife

FOR GOOD FRIENDS AND EXTENDED FAMILY

A similar approach can work with good, but not best, friends. Although you may not want to mention it to those who aren't your very closest friends, consider that there are potential advantages to telling more people instead of fewer. One is you never know who will step up to the plate. Sometimes a friend who was just a good guy you saw around your neighborhood will be the guy who went through it himself last year but never told you. He could have a cousin who is the city's top urologist, or his wife could be a social worker who will hook you up with the best support group. If you give friends a chance to be supportive, they usually are—because that is what friends do for each other.

Sample opener: "I've been having some health problems lately." ("You have? Everything okay?") "I've got prostate cancer. It's not too bad—they caught it early, but Janice and I are still kind of worried."

Introducing the idea that you have some concerns, even if the diagnosis isn't life-threatening, is very important. This lets people know that you could use some help if they feel like offering it. After you admit your worry, it is easy for that friend to say, "Well I've got this cousin who's chief urologist at Metro Hospital. If you want, I could give him a call." If you say, "It's not too bad and I'm sure it'll all be fine," and end there, then your friend will think that you don't really need—or want—any help and, because you're putting the topic to rest, he should not say anything more about it.

FOR CLOSEST FRIENDS AND KEY SUPPORTERS

When you don't feel well, it can be especially difficult to get out of your own head and think of how other people are doing. You might forget how good it feels to be able to do *something* to help a friend in need, even if it is a banal little task. Usually in the face of a friend's hardships, we feel useless and wish there was something we could do. If you need something—a ride to your radiation appointment, a weekend activity to look forward to, or help walking the dog— ask a friend. It's not easy, but you might be surprised how much your friends and family *want* to help you through this, and little practical tasks are an easy way to start.

> "I only told my wife, never told Mom or my kids. The stigma that is attached with this disease. . . I didn't want to deal with it. I know that eventually I will tell, but for now I don't want to worry anyone."
> —Darren N.

For someone you're close to, you don't have to say everything in one conversation. It might be easiest to start slow, simply by telling them about your diagnosis and your reaction. Be patient when waiting for a response: many people feel they don't know what to say to news like this and men especially may tend to respond with silent, but supportive, signals, like a hand on the shoulder or a nod.

Sample Opener: "David, this is hard to talk about, but you and I have gone through a lot together—ever since high school." ("What's going on?") "Well, Janice and I went to the doctor last week, and it turns out I have prostate cancer." ("Oh, no. I'm sorry to hear that.") "Yeah, it looks like I'll have to go through treatment for the next few months…"

If your friend comes out with the standard: "Let me know if there's anything I can do," then make sure you make some positive acknowledgment. You may not feel like you need anything now, but it's smart to leave the door open.

AN IMPORTANT NOTE ON TELLING FAMILY MEMBERS

No matter how private a person you are, you have a responsibility to tell your close male relatives that you have prostate cancer, so that they know their own risk is now elevated. Although the exact role of genetics in this disease isn't clear, prostate cancer does run in families. This is especially crucial when you have been diagnosed with a non-localized cancer at a young age, as most doctors will not routinely screen a man's PSA if he's younger than age 50 (or sometimes younger than age 60). However, in the United States black men should begin screening at age 40.

If you're already through treatment and haven't told someone close to you, it's not too late. It might actually be good timing. At this point, your spouse may be starting to feel stressed out and might be happy if others could pitch in a bit.

Sample Opener: "David, there's been something I've been wanting to tell you. I was diagnosed with prostate cancer a year ago." ("Are you okay? Why didn't you say anything?") "Well, I've gotten through the treatment part okay, but it's really changed things for Janice and me. It's been a tough adjustment. I didn't say anything because I didn't want to worry you . . ."

This can be new territory for a lot of men. For some, the only person they ever share these kinds of details with is their spouse. If talking about these topics with your friends is too difficult, consider talking with men who know all about it in a group meeting for prostate cancer patients. (If the words "support group" bother you, try thinking of it as a meeting where heroic professionals in a challenging field share hard-won knowledge with each other to defeat a common enemy.) Talking in a support group may help you be more willing to reach out to friends or relatives, and you might find that you end up with closer friendships and feel happier and more supported.

It might be better for your marriage, too, if you don't have to rely solely on your spouse for all your support, which could make her feel overwhelmed. Then again, many men also report that leaning on their wives during their cancer experience only made their marriage stronger. Whether or not this is true for you, it's a good idea to gain more understanding of the pressures this illness puts on a marriage and strategies you can use to stay connected.

PROSTATE CANCER RECOVERY AND YOUR RELATIONSHIP WITH YOUR SPOUSE/PARTNER

Whenever a spouse has a health crisis, the dynamic of the relationship can change. Whether the changes in your relationship will be temporary or permanent, for better or for worse, only time can tell. Understanding what's at stake and what you can do to improve things can help you and your partner—and your relationship—survive this experience intact.

Prostate cancer is centered in what could be called the nexus of the male body: where sexual, urinary, and rectal systems—three very private and important functions—all meet. All three of these bodily areas are not simply physical— they are loaded with cultural, social, and personal meanings. For example, the rectal area is considered dirty and a taboo area in most cultures; and the penis and genital region can be the focus of beliefs about fertility, manhood, strength, power, and status. Such heavily loaded ideas can make prostate cancer a very complicated illness for two individuals to deal with; they may not have matching ideas about these topics and they may be too embarrassed to talk about their ideas openly with each other.

We'll begin this section with a discussion of the kinds of changes you may be experiencing, including sexual ones, and end with professional advice on navigating these changes successfully side-by-side with your spouse.

Relationship Changes that can Occur with Prostate Cancer—Other than Sex

Although many men see their temporary or permanent loss of erectile function as the chief change that affects their relationship post-treatment, most researchers would argue that the bigger changes happen—and need to happen—above the belt buckle: in the brain and in the heart.

CHANGING VIEWS OF YOURSELF

Before you were diagnosed with prostate cancer, there were many roles you played in life: roles related to your work (engineer, teacher, regional manager), your family (son, husband, father, uncle), and maybe your hobbies (baseball fan, photographer, runner). Along with a cancer diagnosis, you are handed a whole new role to play: that of a cancer patient. Especially if you haven't gone through a major illness before, this is a difficult adjustment. Part of your role as a cancer patient involves unpleasant things like getting poked and prodded and talking about genitals and continence issues, all while wearing a skimpy paper gown in a dreary examining room. Anyone would feel a little vulnerable in that position.

Getting a cancer diagnosis can also raise the shadow of mortality. If you are fairly young at the time of diagnosis, you may be wondering if you'll skip right past middle age and go straight to being an old man. Or maybe your diagnosis was more serious, for non-localized prostate cancer, and now you're wondering if you will ever meet your grandchildren. You may feel cheated, or angry, or depressed, or all of those.

> "I have a job, a decent house, a family… but this condition makes me feel insecure, vulnerable in my relationship."
>
> —Darren N.

There are several other factors that can change the way you view yourself. One is the actual physical problems (urinary incontinence, ED, and possible rectal issues) that make you feel as if you have lost control of your own body. Wetting yourself can be demoralizing and can make you feel infantilized. Erectile dysfunction may mean a loss of spontaneous sex or even the end of sexual intercourse all together. Even if he's not currently in a relationship, a man may feel like less of a man with the loss of his erections. Masculinity in most cultures is associated very much with virility and with the phallus, which is a powerful symbol of strength and even life itself. Without such tangible evidence as hard, spontaneous erections or the ability to control basic bodily functions, some men may find themselves questioning, *what does it mean to be a man?* This questioning and vulnerability can change the way you behave in general, and toward your partner in particular.

CHANGES CAUSED BY AGING

Layered on top of any perceived losses of power and manhood are changes in other areas that might be happening simultaneously for many prostate cancer patients. This disease is often diagnosed around the same time a man starts feeling the effects of aging, such as diminished muscle strength and increased pants size. Other obvious signs of age like hair loss or grey hair and wrinkles can add to the feeling that you are losing your virility.

> *"[The ED] bothers me more for him, than for me. I wish I didn't have to see him emasculated."*
> —Leah C., Patient's Wife

> *"Despite having two grown kids and four step-kids, I was very bothered by my new lack of fertility. And I was almost 60 at the time!"*
> —Jake T.

Your spouse may also be going through age-related changes. Menopause can be a rollercoaster of hormones, emotions, and physical symptoms for many women. Your wife may also be in transition in terms of her work life—or adjusting to having you join her at home all day during your retirement.

Given that most men get diagnosed with prostate cancer in their sixties, it is likely to hit a man as he winds down his professional life. Work helps give our lives meaning. Life without work can lower confidence in yourself and may even bring on an identity crisis: Who am I if I'm not an engineer/teacher/salesman? What will I do with my life? This can be especially traumatic if you are beginning to see friends pass away—all of a sudden it may seem as if you are closer to the end of life than you ever thought you were. It may seem as if you are less important to the world, but there is at least one person to whom you are still very important: your spouse.

CARETAKING

No matter how easily your treatments proceeded, there will be times, either during or afterward, when your spouse will need to assume a caretaking role. Caretaking can take many forms: providing emotional support after diagnosis, changing dressings after surgery, buying incontinence pads at the store. Taking care of someone who is having health problems can be difficult for both patient and caretaker. The caretaker is usually glad there are practical tasks to be done and ways she can help her loved one, but she will also have moments of feeling overwhelmed or scared and in need of some support herself.

The business of caretaking can upset the balance of a relationship and some-times make it difficult to continue the usual activities of daily living. The more flexible a couple can be in terms of the roles they take with each other, the better; for example, do both feel comfortable being the giver and the taker? In relationships where the roles are more rigid, it can be more difficult to adjust to stressful shifts in the relationship.

If the caretaking responsibilities begin to seem onerous, then you will need to address the issue. Perhaps there is someone else, a relative or a friend, who you could ask to help. Can you and your spouse arrange it so that she has time to herself—and you do, too—either with friends or on your own, so that you can come back to each other more refreshed? Compromises may need to be made on both sides. Even a small gesture of compromise (maybe you feel too tired to cook but can still peel the carrots) can make the other person feel more appreciated. The person who needs the care might consider little things he could do—fixing a leaky faucet or a cup of tea—to make the caretaker feel cared for, too.

TENSION OVER TREATMENT INVOLVEMENT

In her book *How We Survived Prostate Cancer* (*see* the Appendix), Victoria Hallerman describes how her husband presented her with his treatment deci-sions when he told her about his diagnosis and how this set the tone for her feeling unwelcome as part of his treatment team.

> "Any advice for readers? Yeah, have someone that cares about you help make the decision with you about treatment."
> — Walter M.

> "I found comfort in knowing she was there. She attended doctor meetings with me and kept it straight with me. I don't know that I would've gotten as much information if we hadn't gone over it together afterward."
> — Jake T.

Sometimes patient and spouse can have different priorities for cancer treatment. Research has found that patients might compro-mise their long-term survival rate to maintain potency, whereas their partners value survival over every-thing else.[1] Tensions can rise when fears—for loss of life or loss of man-hood—collide. Hopefully, you and your spouse communicated about your feelings from the beginning. Spouses not only give emotional support, but they can also be very beneficial to a patient by providing an extra set of ears and eyes to catch the many important details of medical treatment, such as understanding the medical information, setting up appointments, following up on test results.

SOCIAL LIMITATIONS

Sometimes the limitations imposed by the disease, or the treatment, can place undue stress on a relationship. For example, the daily radiation treatments could be especially taxing if the treatment center is a long distance from home. Also, complications such as incontinence can result in curtailing a couple's social life and travel. Talk about how you and your partner see these limitations; how much do they bother you? Together, brainstorm for ways to resume more of your desired activities while still maintaining your dignity. For example, staying in a short-term rental house or apartment might give you more privacy on vacation than a hotel—and allow you to do laundry if needed. Changing your regular seats at the theater or ballpark to ones closer to the restroom could allow you to keep your subscription. Initiating new social activities that are more doable but still fun is a great way to broaden your horizons and deepen your bond with your partner. A social worker, support group friend, or your doctor might be able to offer coping strategies as well.

ANXIETY/DEPRESSION

Multiple studies have shown that partners become emotionally distressed at higher rates than patients, and women are more likely than men, in general, to develop depression and anxiety. If you know your partner is feeling anxious and scared about your condition, then you may feel you want to protect her by not sharing your own fears. In reality, there can be great comfort for her in knowing that you are together in your fears or losses. Many couples found that by going through every step of the way together, they came through with a closer, more meaningful relationship and were less "down" than they expected because they weren't alone.

Look for signs that depression or anxiety might be affecting your spouse's daily life. Has she withdrawn from her own support network of friends and family? Does she express guilt about your condition or her role in your life? Can you encourage her to continue or resume activities that once gave her joy? If you feel that she is slipping into a real depression and could benefit from counseling, present the idea as a solution to problems *she* sees in her life. For example, "Your boss seems to be really demanding lately. Maybe a therapist would have some ideas about dealing with him so he doesn't give you such a headache." Or, "You've been saying you have trouble sleeping for weeks now; maybe your doctor would be able recommend ways to sleep better." If she seems reluctant to talk to her doctor or go to a therapist, you might suggest going to couples therapy to get your life together back on track. "We're going through so much right now, it would do us both good to talk these things through." A good couples counselor should be able to help address her individual anxiety or depression, and it would take you out of the position of having to "police" her state of mind.

As discussed in the previous chapter, you are also at a higher risk for depression and anxiety during your cancer experience, and your state of mind will definitely impact your spouse. The best thing you can do is to be honest with yourself and your spouse about what you are feeling. Be vigilant about not taking out any anger or anxiety on your partner. Instead, try some of the suggestions in the previous chapter for feeling better, and don't be too proud to get help when you need it.

NAVIGATING THESE CHANGES IN A HEALTHY WAY

It is important to look at how your health issues and, more importantly, your reactions to them, may be affecting your life with your partner. There are some very common patterns: Some men avoid intimate contact with their wives, out of embarrassment or guilt. Some men retreat altogether, isolating themselves because they are scared or in pain. Some men are angry—with themselves, their doctors, or the disease—and take it out on their partners. Other men may drink too much or try to lose themselves in other activities, in an attempt to not feel the unpleasant way they are feeling.

If any of these scenarios sound familiar, then ask yourself some hard questions: Do you avoid touching your wife because you have ED or other problems? Do you ignore her in other ways because you are caught up in your own anxieties? Do you feel down about what you can't do, yet avoid talking about it? Has all sexual activity just stopped without either one of you trying to talk about what's going on? Do you find yourself raising your voice more often than before or slamming doors? Are you drinking more than you used to?

These very human reactions are destructive to your relationship and hurtful to your spouse. They may also be signs of anxiety and depression. One more question to ask yourself: Do you want to change your actions? That is totally your prerogative—you have the power to make healthy decisions, even when you are feeling sick.

Changes in your Sex Life

Many of the problems that plague couples after prostate cancer treatment come from the same cause, according to Leslie Schover (Professor of Behavioral Science at the University of Texas MD Anderson Cancer Center), who specializes in helping couples with sexual and reproductive issues after cancer treatment. She points out that most couples have unrealistic ideas of what their post-treatment sex life will be like and are caught unaware when problems arise. These unrealistic thoughts—like things will be "back to normal" after surgery is over, or that Viagra will enable them to have sex just like an 18-year-old—are often unspoken by the couple and unchallenged by their medical team. These notions can get in the way of resuming sexual intimacy and rediscovering sexual satisfaction with each other after treatment.

In the absence of adequate pre-treatment counseling about sexual side effects, sometimes the best first step for a couple is to acknowledge they need to re-adjust their mindset, grieve their losses, and then move forward. (Later in this section, Professor Schover shares some techniques.) As discussed above, there are many physical changes that pose mental challenges for men with prostate cancer: the loss of the ability to father children through intercourse, the risk of death, and just the fatigue and pain that can accompany treatment. But perhaps no one change after prostate cancer treatment impacts a couple's life more than erectile dysfunction. (Remember Woody Allen thought that his brain was only his second most important organ.)

ERECTILE DYSFUNCTION

After prostate cancer treatment, most men suffer from ED for some length of time. For some, it is a temporary situation, but it is difficult to patiently await the return of your potency: Post-treatment, men may need 2 years to fully recover their erections. During the waiting time, anxiety and frustration may further impede their attempts to regain erectile function. Or, quite simply and sadly, many couples will just stop trying and never really resume sexual activity, even when it is possible. Remember that satisfying sexual intimacy can be more than vaginal penetration—kissing, touching, oral sex and more can bring fulfillment and variety to your partnership. For other men, ED is a permanent or longlasting condition that must be adjusted to. Either way, there are strategies available to help you deal with the problem, but you must seek them out.

According to a 2005 study, about 59% of all men who experience ED after prostate cancer treatment seek medical help to treat the ED.[2] Many men are willing to try oral medication (Viagra, Cialis) to improve their erections, but if those pills fail, fewer are willing to try more invasive methods like intercavernous injections. Even if the interventions help the man successfully achieve erections, most couples discontinue use soon after trying them.[3]

Many couples also discontinue PDE-5 inhibitor pills, even if they, too, are successful. This abandonment may have its roots in a preconceived notion that sex should be natural and spontaneous and a couple shouldn't have to bother with anything like a pill or a shot before sex. (We hope you will forgive us for pointing out that many women spend their reproductive years bothering with

> "What was vital was our lack of communi-
> cation! I didn't know if he was interested or
> not. His libido seemed down. I wasn't sure
> if it was worth the trouble."
> —Leah C., Patient's Wife

daily pills, or even having devices implanted in their sexual organs, to make spontaneous sex possible.) Sometimes each partner assumes the other doesn't want to "bother" having "assisted" sex. Embarrassment keeps one or both of you from protesting—or perhaps you are even relieved in the moment because you are too exhausted to even consider sex.

DECREASE IN LIBIDO

As already noted, prostate cancer can hit a couple as both people are confronting the physical realities of aging. There can be a decrease in libido in both partners for a whole host of reasons. Fatigue, depressed mood, and emotional responses to cancer diagnosis can afflict both people and, even without other sexual problems, lead to a slowing or cessation of sex.[4] Men treated with hormone therapy experience a severe decrease or disappearance of their libidos. While enduring the challenges of prostate cancer treatment, many couples have to simultaneously survive the woman's journey through menopause, whose symptoms can make communication—and sex—more difficult. Both partners may feel alternately guilty about their own lack of interest, or worried about their partner's.

Some couples recommend checking in every few weeks with each other to make sure each partner is still on the same page about wanting or not wanting sex. Partners are often reluctant to raise the subject of sex because they don't want to add to their spouses' embarrassment; each wants to help the other preserve their dignity in the face of demoralizing changes. Silence can lead to distance in a relationship, which leads to increased distress in both partners, which can lead to worse health outcomes for the patient.[5]

There may be a loss of libido on both sides or a strong desire for sexual intimacy on both sides: being sure that you are both feeling the same way can be a huge relief for both of you. If one partner wants to pursue sexual intimacy and the other doesn't, then it will be necessary to discuss compromises. Ignoring your spouse's needs, or getting angry because she doesn't respond to yours, is no way to solve the problem.

A problem may arise if men leak urine when they have sex or during orgasm after prostatectomy. The man may be embarrassed and the partner turned off by its happening. The problem needs to be discussed with your doctor and can be minimized if the man urinates immediately before the couple has sex. (see Chapter 3).

A Patient's Story: Mutual Lack of Libido

In today's hypersexualized world, it may seem like heresy to admit that you're okay with not having sex, but some patients are. This can be especially true of men who were already beginning to notice a decrease in their libido because of aging or other health problems. Reggie M. has been on hormone therapy for advanced prostate cancer for more than 5 years and has severe ED; his wife had already lost her libido when going through menopause and breast cancer years prior and had just endured a recurrence of her breast cancer. "Our marriage has gotten stronger as a result [of our health problems]," said Reggie. "When one party does [want sex] and the other doesn't, then there's trouble, but when this happened to me, it became a level playing field. She isn't frustrated and I'm not frustrated." Reggie reflected, "When I look back on our marriage, there's a lot more than having sex. Just being with her is fulfilling—and 20 years ago, I never could have said that."

How to Find your Way Back to Each Other—Sexually and Otherwise

Both erectile dysfunction and loss of libido can be understandable setbacks in a couple's sex life. But most couples don't want their sex life to end forever. Even during the hiatus of healing, there are things a couple can do to stay connected while waiting to resume sexual intercourse. Professor Leslie Schover suggests several concrete strategies couples can use to improve their chances of marital happiness.

- Couples frequently feel they were not adequately forewarned about potential complications—or they just didn't expect to have any. One of the most important things a couple can do as soon as possible is to *readjust their expectations*. Instead of constantly comparing your current intimacy with your pre-diagnosis sex life, you should focus on the here-and-now. Memories are to be treasured, and the loss of youthful sexual energy is to be mourned, but then it is time to move on to what you can do today. Don't let the ghosts of sex life past get in the way of your present potential.
- Go back to sex with less pressure on performance and more of an attitude of exploration. In her therapy practice with post-cancer couples, Dr. Schover recommends starting with Sensate Focus

Exercises (*see* the Appendix for guides on these exercises) that can give couples a framework for resuming touch without a lot of pressure on sexual performance—these exercises can help you explore what *else* feels good sexually and can lay the foundation for new ideas of intimacy in your relationship.

- Another way to decrease the pressure associated with resuming sex is not to build up your hopes to a big "second honeymoon" when you plan to start trying to have sex again. Such build-up puts a lot of pressure on both partners, and "that's a great way to ruin a vacation," notes Dr. Schover. There are no guarantees that sex will go smoothly the first time (or second, or tenth. . .) after cancer treatment—even with pharmaceutical help. Instead, take mini-vacations and set aside time in a relaxed way to explore each other without the pressure.

- It is important that this new exploration be a joint project. Who usually initiates sex? Often it has been the man's "job" to suggest sex and the woman might not want to put herself out there or might feel rejected because of her man's apparent lack of interest. Both spouses need to make effort if resuming intimacy is important to them.

- Don't stop physically touching each other just because it won't lead to intercourse. A lot of times men don't want to "start something they can't finish" so they stop showing any kind of physical affection. Women miss casual loving touch as much as (sometimes more than) penetrative sex. Men think they are doing women a favor, but really they are creating distance in the relationship. Keep touch alive in the relationship: hug, kiss, hold hands, pinch bottoms, or just cuddle up to watch TV.

Other experts in the field have done studies that support some additional suggestions. For example, both partners need a good support network. Couples with numerous social and psychological sources of support have an increased chance of coping well with the problems thrown their way.[6]And in case we haven't stressed this one enough: communicate. Don't assume you know what your partner is thinking, no matter how long you have been together. The future of your sex life could depend on your willingness to talk about things that are difficult to talk about. Several studies have shown that patients who engage in active cognitive and emotional processing of the cancer experience report lower distress.[7,8]

Together with your partner, explore new ideas about your life together. How do you want to define yourself post-treatment? What activities will give meaning to your life? How do you want to be as a couple? How will you be physical together? How important is it to pursue further treatment to resolve issues like

Gay Partnerships and Prostate Cancer

Prostate cancer poses challenges to every intimate relationship. Although most of those challenges are the same whether the couple is straight or gay (we use the feminine article to refer to spouses in this chapter for reasons of space and easy reading), there are some specific areas of concern for gay men and their partners.

For one thing, a gay male couple has a much higher chance of being affected by this disease because both partners are at risk. Researchers estimate there is a 28% chance of one partner of a gay couple getting prostate cancer during their lifetimes.[i] The estimates are that 2 to 3% of the population is gay or bisexual and that there are 5000 new cases of prostate cancer each year in that population.[ii] Despite the large number of gay men alive with prostate cancer in the US (about 50,000), there are no scientific studies and only three publications that even address the issue.

Sexually, the loss of erectile function could have a different meaning for a gay couple, depending on their sexual activities. The hardness of an erection needed for oral or manual stimulation is much less than that needed for penetrative sex, and some gay couples are more accustomed to these forms of sex and therefore more likely to define sexual intimacy more broadly than some straight couples. On the other hand, stimulation of the prostate gland and anal intercourse are more frequently a part of gay pre-treatment sex life. Surgical removal of the prostate, or radiation damage to the rectum and surrounding area, may directly affect those aspects of a couple's sexual life.

Your doctor may not be very aware of these issues, or may feel uncomfortable talking about them, or he/she may not be so sensitive in bringing them up. If this is the case, or if you just don't feel comfortable talking about intimate matters with your doctor, the Gay Medical Association can help you locate gay-friendly physicians and/or therapists in your area (www.glma.org). A couples therapist who specializes in working with gay couples could also help you and your partner through this time. Some regions offer support groups that focus on the gay cancer experience (or, rarely, specifically prostate cancer). There are also online communities for gay men with cancer, such as Out With Cancer (*see* Appendix).

[i] Couper JW. The effects of prostate cancer on intimate relationships. *Journal Men's Health & Gender*, 2007; 4(3): 226–232.
[ii] Blank TO. Gay men and prostate cancer: invisible diversity. J Clinical Oncology, 2005; 23: 2593–96.

urinary incontinence or ED—to both of you? What activities (physical or not) will add intimacy to your relationship? If you are having trouble opening the discussion, then a couples counselor can help the two of you work through a list of questions like these.

THE ARGUMENT FOR COUPLES THERAPY

There's a common saying about prostate cancer—that it is a couples' disease, not an individual one, because it can so deeply affect a life partnership. It makes sense, then, that one good way of addressing the problems of the couple, and the patient himself, is in couples' therapy. Therapists trained to work with couples specialize in areas of intimacy and communication, so it shouldn't be too difficult to find a professional that could help you work through prostate-related issues. Most couples report having difficulty talking about their sex lives, so if you and your partner have been ignoring the topic, then you are not alone. If making an appointment with a couple's therapist is intimidating, then you could start by sitting down with your treating physician (or your primary care physician) and your spouse for an opportunity to discuss any medical issues among the three of you.

Maybe you're thinking: "To heck with all this talking, all we need is to get rid of this ED and our problems are solved!" Erectile dysfunction often comes as a surprise after treatment; even if they have been forewarned, many men just assume it won't happen to them. Studies have shown that most couples in this situation believed that their sex life would continue as normal after cancer treatment through the use of sexual aids (such as Viagra) rather than through any changes in their sexual practices.[9] Earlier in this chapter we quoted statistics that most couples abandon ED treatments—even when they prove effective. Indeed, one research group reported that only 10% of men were satisfied with their ED treatment.[10] Obviously, there is more at play here than just the need for an erection. Perhaps the dissatisfaction with, and abandonment of, ED treatments points to inadequate mental and emotional preparedness for certain changes in a couple's sex life and what those changes will mean for their relationship. The best solution (barring a magic bullet treatment for ED) would be ample pre-counseling for couples on cancer treatment side effects and lots of sensitive and informed follow-up during and after treatment. For various reasons, that sort of interdisciplinary work is hard to come by in our current medical system, and add to that the fact that many couples have a hard time with the idea of visiting a therapist. What to do?

Luckily, there will be more alternatives to in-person couples counseling available soon: Dr. Schover and others are working on an Internet-based couples therapy specially tailored for prostate cancer survivors and their partners. Preliminary results show that such an intervention can improve men's sexual satisfaction and function. The couples with the best outcomes were ones in whom the male switched to a more intensive ED treatment (Vacuum Erection Device, injections, penile prosthesis) after having only used pills with poor results or having not used any medical treatment before therapy.[11]

If couples therapy isn't doable for you, you might try a support group—for patients, or for spouses (*see* Appendix for more info on finding groups in your area). Another study comparing different therapeutic interventions found that one of the best methods was actually sending the men to 10 weeks of group therapy after their treatment. The focus of the therapy sessions was stress reduction related to the after-effects of prostate cancer.[12] All the men who took part in the therapy showed improvement in their sexual function as well as their stress levels. Let's face it: most doctors (whether cancer docs or primary care docs) do not spend enough time counseling patients on how to deal (emotionally and physically) with ED; you might really benefit from taking the time to hear how others make it through. Your doctor (or his/her office staff) can point you toward a group meeting in your area.

THE DOCTOR–PATIENT RELATIONSHIP

Prostate cancer brings another relationship front-and-center in your life: your relationship with the physician treating your cancer. This can be especially true when you are dealing with side effects after treatment and have to return to the doctor many times. There will surely be moments in your interactions with your doctor that are uncomfortable—to minimize any discomfort, we offer some pointers from the docs themselves.

Doctors are not Offended If You go for a Second Opinion

If you are considering a certain cancer or side effect treatment and can't make up your mind, it is a good idea to get a second opinion from another doctor. Some patients hesitate because they are concerned about how their doctor will feel. You should not worry about offending the first doctor you see, whether or not you end up going back to him for treatment. Good doctors should not be offended—they want you to get care that you are satisfied with.

If the two doctors don't agree in their opinions and you don't know which to trust, you may need to get a third opinion (even if it means traveling to another town) for clarification. Make sure that you are clear with the office staff about your diagnosis and the fact that you are looking for a second opinion when you call a doctor's office for an appointment. Especially if you are calling a prominent doctor, you may be given an appointment date long in the future—the staff will generally be able to adjust this if your diagnosis is one that needs to be acted on quickly.

Doctors Can Feel Uncomfortable Talking About Sex, Too

In an ideal world, we would all be able to find doctors that are a balanced mix of great medical skill and interpersonal sensitivity. In the real world, however, your doctor probably has more of one than the other, and most of us would value medical skill over approachability when it comes to cancer. You might get the feeling that your doctor would rather be doing the actual treatments instead of sitting in his office talking about your sex life. Regardless of whether that is true, studies have shown that patients do not discuss sexual topics with their health-care practitioners if they perceive any discomfort with this topic.[13] By not discussing sexual topics, you and your doctor will miss the opportunity to discuss treating and solving these problems. Although it shouldn't be the patient's responsibility to raise the issue of sexual problems or additional treatment, you may have to initiate the conversation or revive the discussion if your doctor tries to end it prematurely. As awkward as it may feel, persevere until all your questions have been answered.

Doctors may Underestimate your Distress

At least one research study proved that there is often disagreement between the patient's and the doctor's assessment of the patient's distress, with doctors underestimating the severity of the patient's problems.[14] This might be a result of the patient not adequately sharing his concerns or of the doctor not adequately listening. Regardless of blame, it is important that your doctor really understand what is going on with your body and how much it is bothering you. As we noted earlier, the degree of bother caused by a health problem is often a good guide for how aggressively to pursue treatment. One effective solution is to bring your spouse or a friend with you to serve as a "communication conduit" between you and your physician.[15]

Consider Enlarging your Care Team

When involved in a struggle against cancer, you must rely on your treating physician for advice, expertise, and healing. A disease like prostate cancer

A Note to Doctors and Other Medical Care Providers: Ideas to Improve Communication About Sensitive Issues

An excellent 2001 research study analyzed the impact of a couples therapy intervention with men and their spouses who were recovering from prostate cancer. The program focused on enhancing recovery from treatment, improving communication, and restoring intimacy in the relationship. One of the facts the researchers stressed was that patients are not prone to volunteering information about their sex life and need sensitive prompting that is most effective when incorporated into routine health assessments. Although not every medical group can implement a specialized protocol, there were several general conclusions that can be followed by almost any caregiver working with prostate cancer patients and their families.

1. Knowledge of sexual topics and self-awareness about your own attitudes toward these topics can make you more skilled and comfortable in discussing them with your patients. Ideally, your knowledge would encompass sexual mores of the various ethnic and cultural populations you serve. Regular staff debriefings can provide opportunities to share ideas and resources.

2. A sexual history interview guide can provide structure during challenging discussions. Getting the basic sexual history in advance of treatment will also help identify areas of possible concern.

3. Develop and nurture a trusting relationship with both people in the couple. Consider how some very basic aspects of care can show your respect of your patients, like providing a private and comfortable room for these discussions. (And we hope it goes without saying that your cell phone should be off.)

4. Be sure to pay attention to both verbal and non-verbal cues—this can tell you a lot about the couple's relationship and give you clues about feelings that aren't articulated.

5. Be ready to offer information and resources about sexual behavior beyond intercourse. In the face of ED and other sexual side effects, many couples need some help getting creative in their approach to sexuality.[i]

[i]Monturo CA, Rogers PD, Coleman M, Robinson JP, Pickett M. Beyond sexual assessment: lessons learned from couples post radical prostatectomy. Journal of the American Academy of Nurse Practitioners 2001:13;511—516.

affects much more than your prostate and can have serious impact on your mental and relationship health. Ideally, every urologist and oncologist who treats prostate cancer patients would inquire at length about your sexual health and screen patients for depression or anxiety, but that does not usually happen in the real world. Doctors are rushed, embarrassed, or uncomfortable discussing such topics; they may feel them to be too far outside their area of expertise.

If you feel like your health needs aren't being adequately addressed with one doctor, maybe it is time to enlarge your care team. Your physician probably has trusted colleagues in other fields (such as sex therapy or psychiatry) to whom he can refer you. If he doesn't offer, you or your spouse might need to ask; this can be usually done at an appointment or on the phone with a member of the doctor's office staff.

You could also try approaching your primary care doctor for direct help or referrals. Primary care physicians are more accustomed to treating the whole patient and may be better positioned to refer you to professionals who can help you. Some medical practices, particularly those located in hospitals, may have social workers or nurse practitioners on staff to assist you. Don't make the mistake of thinking you are being passed off to less knowledgeable underlings— these professionals often have more experience and time to counsel patients and their families going through cancer treatment than doctors do.

The Future of Prostate Cancer Treatment and Recovery

This chapter will introduce possible future therapies and a new diagnostic test for prostate cancer and the most common side effect of prostate cancer treatment, erectile dysfunction (ED). Also in this chapter, we will give a brief discussion of medical research trials and some factors to consider if you are thinking about volunteering as a study participant.

NEW DIAGNOSTIC TEST

The Prostate Cancer gene 3 (PCA3) is a new marker for prostate cancer that was discovered in 1999. Unlike the Prostate Specific Antigen (PSA), high levels of PCA3 are associated only with prostate cancer, not benign disease. The presence of PCA3 can be measured in urine and the level of PCA3 can help determine how likely it is that prostate cancer is present and when it is necessary to get a biopsy.

The PCA3 test is done after a digital rectal examination (DRE), when cancerous cells with high levels of PCA3 migrate from the prostate into the urine. A urine sample is sent to a laboratory, where a PCA3 score will be assigned (anywhere from 1–125). A high PCA3 score points to an increased likelihood of the presence of prostate cancer cells and would suggest an immediate biopsy. A low PCA3 score means there is a decreased likelihood of a cancer. If the PCA3 score is low enough, a biopsy could be delayed or even avoided all together. By helping doctors determine when it is time to biopsy a patient's prostate, the PCA3 test may help to avoid or delay biopsies. The PCA3 test is currently approved in Europe but not in the U.S. If approved, then this test would (along with various PSA tests) help distinguish between cancerous and non-cancerous prostates, between aggressive and non-aggressive cancers, and help select which patients may need a first or repeat biopsy.

NEW TREATMENTS FOR PROSTATE CANCER

Prostate cancer is one area of medical research that always seems to be thriving. The reasons are obvious: it is a common disease, so the number of people who could be helped is enormous. Also, as evidenced in the previous 10 chapters, the current treatments all leave something to be desired in terms of after-effects. So the search continues, with glimmers of possible success, for treatments that are highly effective, minimally invasive, and cause few side effects.

High-Intensity Focused Ultrasound

High-intensity focused ultrasound (HIFU) is the newest therapy for prostate cancer. As of the end of 2010, HIFU has been approved for use in Europe, Canada, South Korea, and South America but has not yet been approved in the United States as a primary treatment for prostate cancer. (It may be used as a salvage treatment if a patient has a recurrence after radiation.) HIFU is a focused high-energy sound wave, guided by a computer so that it heats and destroys the tissue at a certain focal point at a distance from the ultrasound wand. Thus, the tissue of the rectum is not heated—only the prostate in front of it.

The focused sound waves raise the temperature of the targeted tissue to 65°C to 85°C (149°F–185°F), and the cells of the tissue become coagulated (like an egg in a frying pan) and the cells die. The uniqueness of HIFU is that it can pass deep into body tissue and will heat only a very small area, about 10 mm by 2 mm (two-fifths by one-twelfth of an inch) wide. In that way, the sound wave can pass through the rectal wall without injuring the delicate lining of the rectum. The treatment can be repeated if the first treatment is not successful, with no damage to the unheated tissue. It can also be offered to men whose cancers return after radiation therapy.

The HIFU treatments are done as an outpatient procedure, take about 2 hours (the range is 1 to 3 hours), and are done with the patient anesthetized in an operating room. After anesthesia is given, an ultrasound wand is placed in the rectum. The energy waves transmitted through the probe actually cook and kill small portions of the prostate. A catheter is placed into the bladder before procedure and is kept in for at least 1 week and up to 2 weeks afterwards. The cells of the cooked prostate die and are expelled during urination over the next several months. During that time, the patient will experience some urinary symptoms, including some pain, increased urgency and frequency.

One of the problems with the device is that the beam treats only a region of the prostate: this is great if the small region contains all the cancer cells but not so great if there are some cancer cells elsewhere in the gland. During the procedure, the person controlling the rectal probe that delivers the HIFU, either by hand or by computer, cannot see the cancer. Magnetic resonance imaging (MRI) technology is the only proven method to accurately pinpoint the cancer, but an MRI cannot be used during HIFU treatment because two probes cannot fit (and still work accurately) in the patient's rectum at the same time. The bottom line is that the volume of tissue to which the HIFU energy is delivered is not completely controlled.

There are two models of HIFU devices. One is the Ablatherm, developed in 1989, with which (as of 2010) 21,000 people have been treated. This device is programmed for robotic control of the treatment with a single passage of the probe. The other device is the Sonablate 500, which was developed in the early 1990s for the treatment of benign prostate disease and then modified to treat prostate cancer. The Sonablate is a manually operated system under control by the surgeon, who manipulates the wand to deliver the HIFU. To date, the success rate seems to be a little better with the computer-controlled device, but there is very little data to compare.

Recently, several reviews of HIFU treatment have been reported in the urologic literature.[1,2,3] In one, an effort was made to determine whether the treatment actually cured the cancer and whether it caused problems with urination or erectile function, like surgery or radiation can. Although long-term data is missing for the effectiveness of the treatment, at a 2-year follow-up, only 60% of the men had a reduction in total prostate-specific antigen (PSA) to a level below 0.2 ng/mL. That number should be compared to 88% of men who have a PSA less than 0.2 ng/mL 5 years after radical prostatectomy. Remember that 15 years of follow-up are needed to determine the true effectiveness of a prostate cancer treatment.

Another problem with HIFU is that the prostate volume must be less than 40 g. That excludes about half the patients, or they must first be treated with androgen deprivation therapy (ADT) to shrink the prostate. (*See* Chapter 8 for a discussion of ADT therapy and its side effects.) Other complications include urinary tract infections (which affect about one in four patients), an incontinence rate of 20%, and an impotence rate of nearly 80%. The impotence rate is so high because of the burning of nerves that run close to the prostate. Also for one in three HIFU patients, there is a need for surgical intervention to remove the burned (dead) tissue of the prostate or to correct a stricture of the prostate, bladder neck, or urethra (*see* Chapter 5 for more information on strictures and surgery).

Thus it appears that the quest for an incision-less removal of the prostate is associated with many problems and a less efficacious cure rate than the therapy with an incision. (For those interested in reading about real men's experience with HIFU, *see* the Appendix.)

Cryotherapy

Cryotherapy for the treatment of prostate cancer is a special case—we could have included it in the chapter of accepted therapies because it has long been FDA-approved in the United States. However, the cryotherapy systems in use today are being marketed, based on FDA approval before 1976. In that year, the Medical Device Amendments were applied to the Federal Food, Drug, and Cosmetic Act, requiring important scientific proof of a device's efficacy in the form of clinical trials. As a result of the absence of those trials, we have chosen to place cryotherapy as a possible future treatment.

Cryotherapy is a treatment to kill cancerous tissues with use of extremely cold temperatures. Severe cold can cause the tissue to die through several different mechanisms:

1. The direct effect of the creation of ice crystals in the cells
2. The dehydration of the cells
3. Destruction of blood vessels that feed the tumor
4. The effect of rapidly warming the frozen cells, which makes the cells swell and causes them to malfunction and die

It is important that the tissue be rapidly frozen and thawed for the treatment to be effective. A freezing temperature of −40°C for 3 minutes is thought to be sufficient to eradicate the tumor.[4] The process of freezing and thawing is repeated in two or three cycles to make it more effective.

As with HIFU, cryotherapy is done under anesthesia in the hospital. The technique uses thin needles placed through the perineum (the area between the scrotum and the rectum) into the prostate. The needles are attached to pressurized gas tanks of argon to freeze and helium to thaw. The gas is fed into the needles at lowered pressure, resulting in the creation of the very low temperatures and freezing of tissues.

The proper placement of the needles is observed with an ultrasound probe that is placed into the rectum before the procedure begins (but after the anesthesia). The freezing of the prostate cells can be seen by the doctor in real time on the ultrasound monitor. As with radiation and HIFU, after the treatment is complete, the prostate gland remains in its usual position, so the anatomy is unchanged, and the bladder, prostate, and urethra remain in continuity.

The statistical results of cryotherapy as a primary treatment for prostate cancer are still unclear. So far, there is a lack of agreement between study groups and a mixture of simultaneous therapies (like hormone therapy) are often included in the reports. After cryotherapy, the majority of men are impotent because the ice ball extends to the nerves lying on the surface of the prostate capsule and kills the nerve fibers so that they cannot function. (This might be avoided if only one side of the prostate needs to be treated.) Other possible complications include incontinence caused by destruction of the sphincter and bladder neck, strictures of the prostate, fistula (a hole) between the prostate and rectum, and, of course, lack of cure of the cancer. As with HIFU, there is no long-term data to determine the rate of cure of the cancer by this therapy.

On the positive side, cryotherapy is, like HIFU, a minimally invasive procedure that could be repeated if needed and can be regionalized, meaning it can treat just one side of the prostate if that is where the cancer is confined. In fact some centers use the therapy like a frozen lumpectomy. Because there is no good long term data, it is difficult to decide at this time if its use is wise for the general population.

Photodynamic Therapy

During photodynamic therapy (PDT), a chemical is infused into the patient's blood that, when exposed to specific wavelengths of light, will form a product called reactive oxygen species, which kills cancer cells. Reactive oxygen species are like the bubbles formed from hydrogen peroxide. These scrubbing bubbles are free radicals that interfere with the chemistry of the cell. The reactive oxygen species are only activated by a special laser light, which is directed inside the body into a specific area during PDT. Photodynamic therapy is given under anesthesia and the laser fibers used to deliver the light are placed into the prostate in much the same way that the needles are placed that are used to deliver the radioactive seeds for brachytherapy treatment.

PDT is approved in the United States for treating cancer of the esophagus, small cell lung cancer, and inflammatory disease of the esophagus, but not for prostate cancer. There are ongoing clinical trials of PDT for prostate cancer in Canada and the United Kingdom, but not the United States as yet. The therapy can be given to men who have had radiation whose cancer is still progressing afterward, without danger to the affected tissues. Moreover, it can be given again and again. At this time, the principal interest in its use seems to be as salvage therapy—for men who have had a recurrence after radiation who otherwise have few options for additional treatment—rather than as primary treatment for the disease.[5] In the U.S. study, all of the men who had radiation failures and then pursued PDT had a relapse over time. This treatment will probably not be available in the United States for some time.

Focal Therapy

Focal therapy is not a particular medical mechanism, but, rather, a new approach to prostate cancer care. Focal therapy treats only one area of the prostate where the cancer is, and the immediate margin around the cancer, so as to reduce damage to erectile nerves, blood vessels, and other structures that allow normal urinary control. Focal therapy could use a treatment like HIFU and cryotherapy that can be regionalized to one area of the prostate and thereby have the possibility of giving better results for potency and urinary control than can surgery or radiation.

Similarly to a "lumpectomy" given to women with breast cancer, in which a lump of cancerous breast tissue is removed rather than removing the entire breast, these treatments attempt to cure the cancer while leaving the body basically intact. The problem with treating only one area of the prostate is that in the majority of men, prostate cancer is a "multifocal" disease, meaning that it can arise in many areas of the prostate at the same (or later) times. If you treat only one area and miss another region of the prostate that contains a tiny amount of the cancer, then you are not doing a proper cancer treatment, and the patient is put at risk for cancer progression. So the potential price to pay for the desire to preserve potency and continence could be uncured cancer or even death. To even consider such a choice, a patient should have multiple biopsies of his prostate at very small intervals (5 mm, one-fifth inch) to give a best estimate of the exact location of the disease.

Focal therapy is a feasible alternative for some patients, although not many studies have been done to date, and those that do exist are by single institutions, on small numbers of men, with limited long-term data, and variable methods of describing the extent of disease. The principle of *caveat emptor* (let the buyer beware) prevails in health care: never forget that the price for failure of a new, unproven treatment could be your life. In the case of focal therapy, there is the possibility that a patient could try radiation or surgery as a salvage procedure (should the cancer progress after focal therapy), provided it is not already too late.

FUTURE THERAPIES FOR ERECTILE DYSFUNCTION

Many men who have ED after prostate cancer therapy have tried at least one of the non-surgical therapies to treat that side effect. Those men not satisfied with the results ask, "What else is on the market to help resume sex?" There currently are no other FDA-approved therapies other than those covered in Chapter 4. However, there are some new therapies in the planning stage and some in early clinical trials. Two of the therapies with the most potential include gene therapy and stem cell therapy; nanoparticles is one of the most futuristic.

Nanoparticles to Treat Erectile Dysfunction

A new developing field in medical therapies for ED is with the use of a new technology known as nanoparticles. Nanoparticles are very, very small spheres (one-billionth of a meter), which because of their small size, when applied in a special paste, are able to penetrate the skin and enter the cells deep in the tissues. In one recent report, nanoparticles were combined with the nitric oxide gas (the gas normally released from nerve endings that initiates erection, as shown in Figure 4.2) and placed on the skin of the penis of normal rats. The nanoparticles were able to pass not only through the skin but also into the erectile tissue of the rats, and they caused an erection. This is an exciting development for all men with ED, as erections could be created simply by rubbing a small amount of cream on the penis prior to intercourse. It is a particularly important finding for men with nerve damage after radical prostatectomy, because in those men, the signal to the cells—the release of nitric oxide—is lost because the nitric oxide is usually released from the endings of the nerves, diffusing into the smooth muscle cells to make them relax. The nanoparticles have the potential to directly bypass the nerve release by stimulating the cells with their hosted nitric oxide. Many experiments will have to be performed in animals, and then trials will need to be performed in humans to determine whether it is safe and effective, but the new concept is certainly an exciting one.

STEM CELL THERAPY

Several research groups around the world are evaluating another new potential method of ED (and possibly urinary incontinence [UI]) therapy that would instill human stem cells into various organs to change the interior cellular structure of the penis. The concept that stem cells might improve ED is just beginning to be tested by some researchers.

Stem cells are primitive, undifferentiated cells found in very young embryos, fetuses, and adults. "Undifferentiated" means that the stem cell can literally transform itself into almost any other type of cell found in the body. All of the fuss concerning the medical use of stem cells is related to the use of harvesting the cells from *unused* fetal tissue—that is, from tiny fertilized embryos that were produced for couples to use in *in vitro* fertilization but that were never implanted into a recipient mother. As a result of the harvesting of the stem cells, the embryo is destroyed, and the "right-to-life" lobby is against that use, even if the cells are used to cure human disease and save many lives. That political problem changed in July 2009, when the Obama Administration allowed the first use of fetal stem cells in early stage research to correct paralysis after spinal cord injury.

Because of the politics of using fetal stem cells, most scientists have resorted to using adult stem cells for their research. The difference between adult and fetal stem cells is the fetal cells have the capability of maturing into any cell type in the body. Adult stem cells are similar, undifferentiated cells found in tissues or organs but need chemical manipulation to direct them into becoming a certain kind of cell. The adult stem cells are found in brain, bone marrow, blood and blood vessels, skeletal muscle, skin, teeth, heart, gut, liver, the ovaries, fat, and testis. Usually the cells are in the "sleep" mode in those organs, until they are called on to replace an existing cell that is damaged through disease or injury. Because there are very small numbers of stem cells in those organs, researchers have learned to harvest them from the tissues and reproduce or "grow" them outside of the body. Researchers in many different fields are studying the great potential of stem cells to treat a wide variety of diseases.

Erectile dysfunction is one area in which researchers are looking at the promising possibility of stem cell therapy. Some animal experiments have been done that involved injecting stem cells into the penises of rats with ED, and the ED was corrected after the cells were injected.[6] The reasons for the improvement are not clear yet, as it is not known what specific alterations of the injected cells occurred after injection.

The treatment of stress urinary incontinence (SUI) after radical prostatectomy is another potential area that could be treated through stem cell therapy. Stem cell-derived skeletal muscle precursor cells, alone or in combination with fibroblasts (cells that promote collagen or scar tissue growth), have been considered.[7,8,9,10] There were some initial reports from Europe in which skeletal muscle stem cell injections were used to correct SUI in women.[11,12] Those studies were extended to men with SUI after radical prostatectomy, and a report was published giving glowing results, stating that 41 men were continent, 17 improved, and 5 had no change 1 year after an injection of myoblasts and fibroblasts into the external urethral sphincter.[13,14] Disappointingly, the positive results in those reports have been challenged by other scientists,[15,16] who cite the lack of substantiation by other centers regarding the positive effect of the injections. The bottom line is that the treatment may or may not actually work at this time; we do not know, but there is surely enough evidence to make this a possible area of great interest for continued research.

Gene Transfer Therapy

Gene therapy is the process of inserting a man-made gene into cells of an organ, so that the new gene can direct the cells to correct a specific problem through the manufacture of certain proteins. In the case of ED, the genes are inserted into the smooth muscle cells of the penis and direct the manufacture of Maxi-K proteins that enable the smooth muscle cells of the penis to relax and allow the penis to become erect. The goal is that gene therapy can allow you to have normal, spontaneous erections for many months.

For the past 10 years, I have been involved with the development of gene therapy for the treatment of ED. In 2000, I co-founded a company called Ion Channel Innovations to pursue the goal of proving the effectiveness of that therapy and as a result have a firsthand understanding of the tough road that must be followed to make a new therapy available to the American public. I will use my experience with gene therapy research to inform the discussion of clinical trial participation. But first, let's discuss how gene therapy for ED works.

How Genes Work

You have probably heard of people having a gene for a certain trait—if your sister has blue eyes just like your mother's, then you would say she got the gene for blue eyes from Mom. In reality, it is not as simple as one gene equals Mom's blue eyes.

Each gene is a segment of DNA material located in our cells. DNA is like a set of blueprints for building a person. A gene is any given segment along the DNA strand that gives the instructions to the cell for building a certain protein. Genes live in the nucleus of a cell (which is like the cell's brain), constantly reminding the cell to get busy. Usually the gene tells the cell to produce a specific product—typically, a protein or enzyme that can cause a specific reaction in the body.

Unlike the blue eyes example above, many genes cause things to happen in your body that are not permanent, and they may be things that are invisible to the naked eye (such as relaxing smooth muscle cells). Contrary to common perception, a gene stays the same throughout your life, but some of the proteins it instructs the cell to make may change. For example, genes dictate how much calcium to make for your bones and how much hair to make for your head. As you age, the mechanisms of the genetic instructions for these proteins can wear down and cause a decrease in your bone density and an increase in your bald spot.

How Gene Therapy Works

Sometimes diseases arise because of a genetic abnormality that is present at birth. This can include a person having too few genes of a certain type, or too many, or simply genes that do not function as they should. (Examples of such diseases include cystic fibrosis, muscular dystrophy, Tay-Sachs disease, and sickle cell anemia.)

During gene transfer therapy, doctors add a test tube-manufactured gene back into the patient's body that will correct diseases that have not been successfully, or easily, resolved by other means. The man-made gene added into the nucleus of the cell will direct the cell to make a specific protein. There may be less of the protein in the body because of disease or aging, or the gene normally present in the cell may make an abnormal protein.

Although gene transfer therapy as a scientific idea has been around since the 1970s, there have been limited FDA-approved uses of it to date. However, scientists around the world are now pursuing gene therapy as a potential cure for everything from color-blindness to HIV. As attractive as the idea is to patients, the advance of gene therapy (and its approval by the FDA) has been delayed because of some difficulties with earlier gene therapy trials (not for ED) caused by the continued discussion by political, religious, and scientific leaders over whether genetic therapy is actually "playing God." I, for one, don't believe that God wants people to suffer if humans, through medical science, can prevent it. Erectile dysfunction may seem like a minor disease, but I know that it can cause great suffering in a person's spirit, relationship, and heart, and I'm driven to offer men a better solution to this pervasive problem.

How Gene Therapy for Erectile Dysfunction Works

The use of gene transfer for ED caused by prostate cancer treatment is a little different than for genetic diseases. In this case, it is a cancer treatment (radical prostatectomy or radiation) that causes the problem rather than a genetic defect. There is damage to the smooth muscle cells of the penis or the nerves that cause erection. The idea of gene transfer is appealing because one, or only a few, treatments would be needed at long intervals—like twice a year (without the need of other medications)—to achieve the goal of erections that work as spontaneously as those you had before cancer treatment.

The gene that we have used in clinical trials for ED is called the *Maxi-K* gene. It is present in nearly all cells in the body but is especially important in smooth muscle cells because it helps to control whether or not the smooth muscle cells are contracted or relaxed. In the penis, when those cells are contracted, they are also shortened, making the penis flaccid (no erection). When they are relaxed, they stretch out and allow the erectile chambers to fill with blood and the penis becomes erect. For erections to happen, a gene must tell the cell to make Maxi-K potassium channel that allows smooth muscle cells in your penis to relax. This causes an erection to happen in the presence of a sexual signal.

The goal of our gene transfer therapy is to put the *Maxi-K* gene into the smooth muscle cells so it can direct the cells to constantly manufacture the new protein, the Maxi-K potassium channel. When the potassium channel protein is made, it exits the cell and attaches to the outer cell membrane. When the proper sexual signal comes along (down from the brain via the nerves), the newly made potassium channel goes from the closed position to an open one. The open channel causes a cascade of events that make the smooth muscle cell relax, and the man's penis becomes erect. Best of all, when this occurs, it does so naturally. You do not have to plan to take a pill, or inject yourself to have sex: spontaneity can return to your sex life. These results can last for up to 6 months after a single injection of the gene.

The transfer itself is done by a doctor who injects the gene, which is dissolved in a sugar-based solution, into the penis. The injection is totally painless, according to the 20 men who participated in the therapy's Phase I trial. When injected, the gene-containing solution enters the corporal bodies of the penis, crosses the cellular lining, and enters the smooth muscle cells. It is possible that the gene also enters the nerves and blood vessel cells of the penis, but the smooth muscle relaxing effect need only happen in the smooth muscle cells to achieve erection.

The penis is an especially advantageous part of the body to try gene transfer therapy. Because the penis hangs on the outside of the body, it is easily accessible and easy to isolate from the rest of the body. Placing a soft silicone ring around the base before the injection limits the possible spread of the gene to other organs. (The ring is left on for 30 minutes after the injection—none of the study participants complained of pain.) The smooth muscle cells of the penis form a continuous layer of cells, linked together in such a way that allows for easy transfer of the proteins that control relaxation and contraction of the cells. Like a line of dominoes, the protein passes from cell to cell, spreading the word to relax those smooth muscles. The result is a strong erection like those you had pre-prostate cancer.

THE CURRENT STATE OF GENE THERAPY FOR
ERECTILE DYSFUNCTION

In 2008, we completed a Phase 1 safety trial with 20 men using *Maxi-K* gene transfer therapy.[17,18] The trial was done without administering a placebo (a placebo is not necessary until Phase II trials, *see* below), so each participant received a single dose of the gene. The dose of the gene was increased in the subsequent groups to test for safety in higher doses.

A NOTE ON SAFETY

The method used to add the gene to the cells during gene therapy is very important. Part of what determines how the gene is added is the disease being treated. If the disease is a cancer, then each and every cancer cell needs to be treated with the gene that is designed to kill or stop the cancer cell. To accomplish that goal, the gene is attached to a virus and the virus acts as a "carrier pigeon," passing into the cell and bringing the gene into the cell nucleus. The viruses used are live, so it is possible that, for example if the virus that is used is the common cold, then the body could have an immune response to it and reject the virus from doing its job. Some types of virus permanently bind the gene to the chromosome and so the virus and the gene both get copied when the cell divides. That copying of the virus can trigger other unintended and dangerous consequences, such as bodily rejection of the new gene or even a new disease or cancer.

However, if only a few cells need to include the new gene, as is the case when ED is being treated, then another type of "carrier pigeon" is used to escort the gene into the nucleus of the cell—one that is much safer than a virus, called a plasmid or naked DNA. This safer approach, is used for our trials using gene transfer for ED.

The most important result of the Phase I trial was that this treatment seemed safe. That is, there were no serious short- or long-term (up to 4 years) transfer-related side effects or other adverse effects. There was no evidence that the gene was incorporated into the semen. That means that the gene transfer could be done without fear of it having an effect on the man's sexual partner or potential child. (Of course, after radical prostatectomy, that would not be an issue because there is no semen produced.) In the men who responded with improved erections after transfer, the response lasted for 6 months. This matches the earlier results in animal trials.

With the exception of our Phase I trial noted above, there currently are no other open trials that use gene transfer for the treating ED. Based on the positive results of the Phase I trial, Ion Channel Innovations is planning to extend to a Phase II trial that will include more participants and test the therapy against a placebo.

Other researchers are at earlier pre-clinical (animal testing) stages of using gene transfer as a potential therapy for ED. Several groups have conceived of the idea of correcting the nerve damage that can occur during prostate cancer surgery. The idea is to place genes that promote nerve growth in injured nerves either in the penis or as a solution over the area of the nerve injury.[19,20,21] In the animal research, the results have been reduction of the ED, but no human trials have begun to test the waters.

PARTICIPATING IN A CLINICAL TRIAL FOR A NEW THERAPY

It is clear from the letters I receive that many men are not helped by or not satisfied with available therapies and are avidly seeking new methods for help. Here are some e-mails I have received from around the country:

1. *I read about your work with gene therapy treatment for ED. I had a radical prostatectomy in 2001. I am 65 and I have pretty good results with Cialis. However, your treatment looks much better.*

2. *I am a male of 56 years with extreme ED. I can't use oral solutions as each one gives me a severe headache for sometimes days later. This has reduced intimacy with my wife to once a month (sometimes less), as I don't want the pain. Repetitious injections (Tri-Mix, Alprostadil) are costly and painful.*

3. *I had a laparoscopic radical prostatectomy in November 2002. My PSA remains undetectable. I am continent. However, although my surgeon said my surgery was "textbook" nerve-sparing procedure, I have not had return of erectile function. I have tried Viagra, Levitra, and Cialis. I get some "puffiness" but not a full erection. And, of course, they have side effects. I have used a vacuum pump, but the rings are painful, and it's difficult to manage. I have used bi-mix [ICI], and I can have a good erection with an injection. But the spontaneity is gone. Recently, I have been seriously contemplating an implant. But then I read of your research in gene therapy to treat ED, and I hesitate to take this step when something much better may be just around the bend.*

4. *Any information or insight you might have would be welcome. I think what you are doing is wonderful, and if I can be part of it in any way, I would gladly volunteer.*

5. *I've been researching the development of Maxi-K and curiously waiting for its introduction and availability to consumers. Would you please share this product's anticipated availability date for those of us experiencing ED. Also, is it at all possible that I may participate in your clinical trials of Maxi-K?*

Each of the men above have ED after prostate cancer care and are unhappy with the current therapy to the point of requesting to join a clinical trial for a product that has not yet been approved by the FDA for physicians to prescribe to their patients. People want to enter trials because other treatments have failed, and they are desperate to return to normal and be cured of their disease.

The Phases of a Clinical Study

All of the treatments described in this chapter—and the rest of this book—have gone through careful testing before becoming available to a patient population. In the United States, the federal government's Food and Drug Administration oversees the approval of new medical treatments. To get FDA approval, the new therapy, be it a new drug or other treatment, must go through a rigorous testing process that first (and above all) shows that the product is safe and second that it works—that is, the result is what it is advertised to do. It is important for all persons who want to enter clinical trials that they understand the purpose of these trials, how they are done and what information they should receive before they put their bodies on the line.

The testing process for approval is a standard one consisting of three phases, with some special requirements for studies involving ED and other sexual problems. (In July 2009, I was a member of a group at the Third International Consultation for Sexual Medicine that summarized the appropriate guidelines for safety testing. I have borrowed heavily from the summary put together by that group.)

Phase I
In a Phase I clinical trial, a new drug or treatment is tested in a small group of people for the first time with three goals:

1. To evaluate its safety
2. To determine a safe initial dosage range for subsequent studies
3. To identify commonly occurring side effects

Prior to any human trials, extensive experiments must be done in animals (usually rats) to prove that the drug or treatment is safe to use and that it works to cause the intended effect. In this case, we had to prove that gene therapy caused erections in impotent rats before we could undertake the Phase I study on humans. Because Phase I studies are often the first in humans, particular care is spent in designing the study to ensure patient safety. The study must be designed to meet the three objectives, while including recognition of all potential risks, monitoring for those risks, and maintaining adequate precautions to manage those risks.

PHASE II

In Phase II trials, the tested drug or treatment is given to a larger group of people (anywhere from several dozen to several hundred persons) to characterize its preliminary efficacy and to provide additional safety data.

The key objective of the Phase II program is to explore a wide range of doses so as to accurately define the lowest effective dose, the best dose to be used in larger Phase III trials, the maximum tolerated dose, and the dose(s) at which obtrusive side effects appear.

PHASE III

Phase III trials provide the bulk of the "substantial evidence" toward government regulatory approval. All Phase III trials in sexual dysfunction should be randomized, double-blinded, and placebo-controlled. Placebo-controlled means that some men in the trial will not receive the actual agent. They will be *randomly* selected to receive the actual product or a placebo (e.g., a sugar pill solution that looks like the real thing but has no effect). Use of a placebo is very important because of the placebo effect. Because people want to believe that a treatment will work, as many as 30% of those who receive the placebo in a clinical trial will report a positive effect on their health. To determine whether a new therapy really works, patients who receive the actual product must be compared to those who received placebo, and those results must be rigorously evaluated to prove that the drug provides a better response. New treatments are not approved by the government without placebo-based trials. "Double-blinded" means that not only do the patients participating in the study not know whether they are receiving the drug or the placebo, but the researchers also don't know. (Usually a pharmacist or mid-level staff member who has no stake in the outcome tracks who's getting which treatment until the end of the study.) This is to ensure that they do not influence the patient reports, even unconsciously.

Patient Protections: Informed Consent and Institutional Review Boards

Some new medical treatments truly seem like science fiction, but it is important to know that their clinical trials exist in the real world, governed by rule of law and set up in such a way as to provide protection for the people who take part in them. The two most essential safeguards that must be part of any medical experiments are the process of informed consent and the existence of an Institutional Review Board (IRB).

INFORMED CONSENT

An important component of any clinical trial, whether it is Phase I, II, or III, is the use of a proper informed consent. The informed consent is a document that is given by the group conducting the trial to the trial participants. By federal law, every person who enters a trial must sign the informed consent before beginning treatment. The consent must be written in simple language that is understandable to non-medical or scientific persons. If it is not understandable, then it is your obligation to ask questions of the person who is conducting the study until you fully understand. It is the researcher's duty to answer all your questions and make sure they provide clear information—that is not misleading—for participants at any point during the study. The informed consent must be approved by a protective group known as an Institutional Review Board (IRB) or Independent Ethics Committee (IEC).

INSTITUTIONAL REVIEW BOARD

An IRB is designated to approve, monitor, and review biomedical and behavioral research involving humans, with the aim to protect the rights and welfare of the subjects. In the United States, FDA and Health and Human Services regulations have empowered IRBs to approve, require modifications in, or disapprove research or study designs. An IRB ensures that research conducted on human subjects is *scientific, ethical*, and *adheres to safety regulations.*

In the United States, IRBs are governed by the Federal Research Act of 1974, which defines IRBs and requires them for all research that receives funding—directly or indirectly—from the federal government. The idea of an IRB was developed in direct response to research abuses earlier in the twentieth century, such as the Tuskegee Syphilis Study, an unethical and scientifically unjustifiable project conducted between 1932 and 1972 by the U.S. Public Health Service on poor African-American men in rural Alabama.

As required by Federal Law:

1. The IRB must have at least five members.
2. The members must have enough experience, expertise, and diversity to make an informed decision.

3. If the IRB works with studies that include vulnerable populations, then the IRB should have members who are familiar with these groups.
4. The IRB should include both men and women, as long as they aren't chosen specifically for their gender.
5. The members of the IRB must not be all of the same profession and must include at least one scientist and at least one non-scientist.
6. The IRB must include at least one person who is not affiliated with the institution conducting the study or in the immediate family of a person affiliated with the institution. These are commonly called "Community Members."
7. IRB members may not vote on their own projects.
8. The IRB may include consultants, but only actual IRB members may vote.

Final Advice: Proceed with Caution and Temper your Hope

In the United States, most studies of drugs or gene therapies are sponsored—paid for—by for-profit drug companies. The sponsor may officially be conducting the study, but usually the management of the study is transferred to a company known as a contract research organization (CRO). The CRO in turn subcontracts the work to one or more clinical testing sites. Each of those sites has one or more primary investigators. These must be independent physicians who have no financial involvement with the outcome of the research and are legally responsible for making sure the study follows FDA rules. The primary investigator is assisted by one or more clinical coordinators—usually nurses—who are responsible for the day-to-day follow-up. Although the primary investigator's motivation is usually to advance science and medicine, the CRO pays the investigation site based on the number of subjects tested. Therefore, if you are considering taking part in a clinical trial, it is very important that you not allow yourself to be swayed by seductive marketing. Be sure you understand which phase the clinical trial is in and that you know the outcome, in terms of safety issues, of earlier trials if it is a Phase II or III trial.

Many potential clinical trial participants misunderstand the basic purpose of a clinical trial. The goal of all clinical trials is first to show safety and second to show that the treatment works. *The primary benefit, particularly of gene transfer and stem cell research at this early stage, is for societal rather than individual benefit, and that must be emphasized in both the written informed consent and any verbal communication with the patient.* If you are considering taking part in a clinical trial to try a new drug or treatment, ask a lot of questions, discuss it with your own doctor, and carefully evaluate all your options before signing up (For more information on finding clinical trials, see the Appendix.).

There are several reasons that a person might want to be part of a clinical trial; most commonly, he has a disease for which no other therapy has proven effective and he feels he has nothing to lose. Another person might fear his children might one day face the same problem and wish to invest in a future cure. Also, in the United States, all trials are administered free-of-charge to participants, so lack of decent insurance could also spur someone to be a "guinea pig" for science. Whatever your reasons for considering trial participation, you should go into it with your eyes open– and knowing that you might be helping yourself but are most definitely helping the men who will follow you through prostate cancer and its aftermath.   🖋

SUMMARY

The promising new therapies discussed in this chapter are a clear response to the problematic complications of current treatment detailed in the rest of the book. Prostate cancer care can leave a man dealing with side effects that hit him where it hurts—side effects that can deeply impact his quality of life.

The good news is the many medical developments of the recent past made the last decade an exciting one for the treatment of prostate cancer in the United States: for the first time since records have been kept, the reported annual death rate from the disease showed a decrease. That reduction is a direct result of improved early diagnosis because of PSA testing, combined with improved methods of biopsy, and earlier treatment delivered at a time when the disease is curable because it has not yet spread from the confines of the prostate. The beneficiary of those advances is you as the patient and every man with the potential for developing prostate cancer.

Treatments for the side effects of prostate cancer therapy have advanced as well. Artificial urinary sphincters, PDE-5 inhibitors, and others can bring beneficial changes to the lives of prostate cancer survivors. The latest hormonal therapies, although still rife with unpleasant side effects, quite simply add years to the lives of men with advanced disease. We are now at a stage of development of new methods (such as gene and stem cell therapy) that in the future may prove less invasive and more effective, while allowing for more natural bodily function and even better quality of life post-treatment.

RESOURCES

General Prostate Cancer

Peter T. Scardino & Judith Kelman, 2010. *Peter Scardino's Prostate Book, Revised Edition: The Complete Guide to Overcoming Prostate Cancer, Prostatitis, and BPH.* Avery/Penguin Group (New York). Provides a good general overview of the topic.

Stephen Strum & Donna L. Pogliano, 2005. *A Primer on Prostate Cancer: The Empowered Patient's Guide.* The Life Extension Foundation (Hollywood, FL). A very detailed and useful book.

Eric Klein, 2009. *The Cleveland Clinic Guide to Prostate Cancer* (Cleveland Clinic Guides) [Paperback] . Kaplan Publishing (New York). A concise book from the leading hospital for Urology.

http://www.pcf.org Prostate Cancer Foundation's site—good info on recent research and they offer a monthly newsletter. (Last accessed 1/31/11)

http://www.prostatehealthguide.com. Prostate Health Guide—covers prostate cancer and other prostate conditions. (Last accessed 1/31/11)

http://prostatecancerinfolink.net/. From the Prostate Cancer International, a non-profit. Features research news and social networks, including groups for "Wives and Partners" and "ED and Incontinence." (Last accessed 1/31/11)

Similar site en espanol: http://cplatinoamerica.wordpress.com/ (Last accessed 1/31/11)

http://www.mayoclinic.com/health-information/ Reliable general health and prostate cancer information. (Last accessed 1/31/11)

http://well.blogs.nytimes.com/tag/jennings/. Dana Jennings blogs for the New York Times about his experiences with a particularly aggressive form of prostate cancer. (Last accessed 1/31/11)

Clinical Trials

http://www.cancer.gov/clinicaltrials. Find cancer-related trials and read results (Last accessed 1/31/11)

http://clinicaltrials.gov/. Registry of federally and privately supported clinical trials conducted in the United States and around the world. (Last accessed 1/31/11)

Coping

Frank J. Penedo, Michael H. Antoni, & Neil Schneiderman, 2008. *Cognitive-Behavioral Stress Management for Prostate Cancer Recovery Workbook*. Oxford University Press (New York).

Arthur Frank, 2002, *At the Will of the Body:Reflections on Illness*. Mariner Books, (New York). A more scholarly narrative about learning to cope with a changed state of health—Frank had a heart attack and got prostate cancer while still an active, fairly young man.

http://www.cancercare.org/ or 1-800-813-HOPE. Cancer Care is a nonprofit organization that can provide support group information, financial support, and educational workshops for people with cancer and their families. (This website also has a Spanish-language version http://www.cancercare.org/espanol/.) (Both sites last accessed 1/31/11.)

http://www.cancer.org/Treatment/SupportProgramsServices/. The American Cancer Society can help you find support groups, lodging, rides to treatment, educational products, as well as providing an online forum. Their "Man to Man" program is specially tooled for prostate cancer patients and offers one-on-one visits with a prostate cancer survivor, a monthly newsletter, and more. (Last accessed 1/31/11) For more information on "Man to Man" go to:http://www.cancer.org/Treatment/SupportProgramsServices/man-to-man or call 1-800-227-2345.

Doctor–Patient Communication

Jerome Groopman, 2007. *How Doctors Think*. Mariner Books (New York,). Easy-to-read book that gives an overview of doctor-think by a doctor-writer.

prostatecancerblog.net. Leah Cohen, wife of a prostate cancer patient and interviewee for this book, writes this blog "to build bridges between doctors and patients by providing a forum for communication." (Last accessed 1/31/11)

Consumer Reports Health Website also offers some (advertising-free) information on doctors, hospitals, and communication. http://www.consumerreports.org/health/doctors-hospitals/doctors-and-hospitals.htm (accessed 1/31/11)

Future Therapies

http://www.ionchannelinnovations.com/. Dr. Melman's site on gene therapy for ED (Last accessed 1/31/11).

groups.yahoo.com/group/hifu survivors/join. Offers information from men who have undergone HIFU therapy. (Last accessed 1/31/11)

Spouses/Families

Victoria Hallerman, 2009. *How We Survived Prostate Cancer: What We Did and What We Should've Done New Market Press* (New York). One couple's story of diagnosis, treatment, and recovery from the wife's point of view.

Women against Prostate Cancer: http://www.menshealthnetwork.org/wapc/. A group for women to get involved in prostate cancer health Features information on prostate cancer and sexuality to be given to patients and their partners before treatment. (Last accessed 1/31/11)

Us Too (www.ustoo.com) Support groups (online and in person) for families and partners, solid information for all, including written and audio information for sharing with groups or non-internet-literate folks. (Last accessed 1/31/11)

http://www.ladies-prostate-forum.org/ladies/. An online forum for women only (Last accessed 1/31/11)

http://www.hisprostatecancer.com/. An excellent site, addressed to women, but features information on sexuality and support groups that could be useful to men as well—including instructions on sensate focus exercises and readers' stories of sexual recovery. (Last accessed 1/31/11)

National Family Caregivers Association http://www.nfcacares.org Great information on practical resources and grief.

(Last accessed 3/11/11)

ERECTILE DYSFUNCTION AND SEXUALITY

Saving Your Sex Life: A Guide for Men with Prostate Cancer by Dr. John Mulhall—"sexpert" at Memorial Sloan Kettering Cancer Center. Hilton Publishing (Munster IN, 2008). Highly recommended by patients for complete information on post-treatment sexuality.

Impotence Anonymous and I-ANON. Call 1-800-669-1603 for information on local support groups.

sexhealthmatters.org. Website of the *Sexual Medicine Society of North America*. Referrals to ED specialists and general information on ED. (Last accessed 1/31/11)

http://www.sda.uk.net. *Sexual Advice Association, UK.* They have good "fact sheets" on various subjects relating to prostate cancer and ED (click on Advice link at top). (Last accessed 1/31/11)

http://www.prostatepointers.org/mailman/listinfo/pcai. The Prostate Cancer and Intimacy listserv sponsored by prostatepointers.org (part of UsToo). Discussion group for people who are struggling with relationship and sexual problems after treatment for prostate cancer. Note: you must join to see this group, but it is a free membership. (Last accessed 1/31/11)

Libby Bennett & Ginger Holczer, 2010. *Finding and Revealing Your Sexual Self: A Guide to Communicating about Sex* Rowman & Littlefield Publishers, Inc. (Lenham, MD:) Offers simple tools for communicating about sex with your partner.

Barbara Keesling, 2006. *Sexual Healing: The Complete Guide to Overcoming Common Sexual Problems.* Hunter House Publishers (Alameda, CA). Not prostate-cancer-specific, but provides a solid overview of sexual health issues, including detailed instructions on sensate focus exercises.

There are also DVDs available (such as "A Heterosexual Couples Guide to Sexual Pleasure" and "Gay Male Couples Guide to Sexual Pleasure") that visually demonstrate sensate focus exercises.

GAY MEN AND PROSTATE CANCER

http://www.glma.org/. Gay-Lesbian Medical Association. Find a gay-friendly provider and read about health issues that impact the gay community. (Last accessed 1/31/11) http://www.malecare.com/ . A site for gay men with cancer, including information on support groups for gay men and a lot of practical advice. (Last accessed 1/31/11)

Gerald Perlman and Jack Drescher (eds), 2005 *A Gay Man's Guide to Prostate Cancer* (*Journal of Gay & Lesbian Psychotherapy* Monographic "Separates"). Informa Healthcare (London). A book for patients, families, and doctors.

http://www.outwithcancer.com/. A site for gay men and women with cancer that features forums, blogs, online support groups, news, and events. (Last accessed 1/31/11)

Osteoporosis

http://www.boneandcancerfoundation.org/pdfs/prostate-cancer-qa.pdf. Preventing Osteoporosis and information on Bone Metastases from the Bone and Cancer Foundation (Last accessed 1/31/11)

Nutrition

The Prostate Cancer Foundation website (http://www.pcf.org/) has an informative section on Nutrition and Wellness, under "Understanding Prostate Cancer" (Last accessed 1/31/11)

http://www.cspinet.org/. Center for Science in the Public Interest has a great, advertisement-free food information and a monthly nutrition newsletter (general, not pca-specific). The September 2009 issue highlighted Prostate Cancer nutrition. (Last accessed 1/31/11)

There are also several reputable books on nutrition and cancer in general, including:

Abby S. Bloch, Barbara Grant, Kathryn K. Hamilton, Cynthia A. Thomson (eds), 2010. *American Cancer Society Complete Guide to Nutrition for Cancer Survivors: Eating Well, Staying Well During and After Cancer* (American Cancer Society).

Jeanne Besser, Kristina Ratley, Sheri Knecht, Michele Szafranski, 2009. *What To Eat During Cancer Treatment: 100 Great-Tasting, Family-Friendly Recipes to Help You Cope* (American Cancer Society).

Rebecca Katz & Mat Edelson, 2009. *The Cancer-Fighting Kitchen: Nourishing, Big-Flavor Recipes for Cancer Treatment and Recovery.* (Celestial Arts).

Hospice Care (End-of-Life issues)

http://www.hospicenet.org/ This site can help patient and family think out end of life issues and find appropriate care. (Last accessed 1/31/11)

http://www.newyorker.com/reporting/2010/08/02/100802fa_fact_gawande. This article, "Letting Go," by writer and physician Atul Gawande, which appeared in the New Yorker on August 2, 2010, should be required reading for every American, whether faced with dire prognosis or not. (Last accessed 1/31/11)

http://www.aarp.org/relationships/grief-loss/ The AARP's site on grief, loss, and coping strategies. (Last accessed 3/11/11.)

Peyronie's Disease

http://www.PeyroniesSociety.org/. Includes newest information from research and a discussion forum. (Last accessed 1/31/11) http://www.peyronies.org/ A less substantial site, but does includes a forum to share your experiences and read others'. (Last accessed 1/31/11)

RECTAL ISSUES

ICON Health Publications, 2010. *Rectal Bleeding — A Medical Dictionary, Bibliography, and Annotated Research Guide to Internet References.* An in-depth resource guide for medical professionals and interested patients.

NOTES

Chapter 1

1. Jemal A, Siegel R, Ward E, & Xu J. Cancer statistics, 2010. *CA Cancer J Clin.* 2010; 60(5):277–300.
2. Krumholtz JS, Carvalhal GF, Ramos CG, Smith DS, Thorson P, Yan Y, et al. Prostate-specific antigen cutoff of 2.6 ng/mL for prostate cancer screening is associated with favorable pathologic tumor features. *Urology* 2002; 60(3): 469–473.
3. Brawley OW, Gansler T. Introducing the 2010 American Cancer Society prostate cancer screening guideline. *CA Cancer J Clin* 2010; 60(2): 68–69.
4. Zhu H, Roehl KA, Antenor JA, & Catalona WJ. Biopsy of men with PSA level of 2.6 to 4.0 ng/mL associated with favorable pathologic features and PSA progression rate: a preliminary analysis. *Urology* 2005; 66(3): 547–551.
5. Chabanova E, Balslev I, Logager V, Hansen A, Jakobsen H, Kromann-Andersen B, et al. Prostate cancer: 1.5 T endo-coil dynamic contrast-enhanced MRI and MR spectroscopy-correlation with prostate biopsy and prostatectomy histopathological data. Eur J Radiol 2010 doi:10.1016/j.ejrad.2010.07.004.

Chapter 2

1. Kundu, SD, Roehl KA, Eggener SE, Antenor JV, Han M, & Catalona WJ. Potency, Continence, and Complications. *J Urol* 2004; 172: 2227–2231.
2. Parker, Chris. Active surveillance: towards a new paradigm in the management of early prostate cancer. Lancet Oncol 2004; 5: 101–106.
3. Amy S. Duffield, Thomas K. Lee, Hiroshi Miyamoto, H. Ballantine Carter and Jonathan I. Epstein. Radical prostatectomy findings in patients in whom active surveillance of prostate cancer fails. J Urol 2009; 182: 2274–2279.
4. Ian Thompson and Klotz, L. Active surveillance for Prostate cancer. JAMA 2010; 304: 2411–2412.
5. Pathologic outcomes of candidates for active surveillance undergoing radical prostatectomy. Urology 76: 689-692, 2010.
6. Krakowsky Y, Loblaw A, and Klotz L. Prostate cancer death of men treated with initial surveillance: clinical and biochemical characteristics. J Urol 2010; 184: 131–135.
7. Berryhill R, Jr., Jhaveri J, Yadav R, Leung R, Rao S, El-Hakim A et al. Robotic prostatectomy: a review of outcomes compared with laparoscopic and open approaches. *Urology* 2008; 72(1): 15–23.

8. Kundu et al. *J Urol* 2004; 172: 2227–2231.
9. Incrocci L, Slob AK, & Levendag PC. Sexual (dys)function after radiotherapy for prostate cancer: a review. *Int J Radiat Oncol Biol Phys* 2002; 52: 681–693.
10. Sanda MG, Dunn RL, Michalski J, Sandler HM, Northouse L, Hembroff L, et al. Quality of Life and Satisfaction with Outcome among Prostate-Cancer Survivors. *New Engl J Med* 2008; 358: 1250–1261.
11. Bergman J, Kwan L & Litwin M. Improving decisions for men with prostate cancer translational outcomes research. *J Urol* 2010; 183: 2186–2192.

CHAPTER 3

1. Arai Y, Aoki Y, Okubo K, Maeda H, Terada N, Matsuta Y, et al. Impact of interventional therapy for benign prostatic hyperplasia on quality of life and sexual function: a prospective study. *J Urol* 2000; 164(4): 1206–1211.
2. Incrocci et al., *Int J Radiat Oncol Biol Phys* 2002; 52: 681–693.
3. Montorsi F, Brock G, Lee J, Stief C. Effect of nightly versus on-demand vardenafil on recovery of erectile function in men following bilateral nerve-sparing radical prostatectomy. *European Urol* 2008; 54: 924–931.
4. Raina R, Agarwal A, Ausmundson S, Lakin M, Nandipati KC, Montague, et al. Early use of vacuum constriction device following radical prostatectomy facilitates early sexual activity and potentially earlier return of erectile function. *Int J Impot Res* 2006; 18, 77–81.
5. Köhler TS, Pedro R, Hendlin K, Utz W, Ugarte R, Reddy, P et al. A pilot study on the early use of vacuum erection device after radical retropubic prostatectomy, *BJU Int* 2007; 100: 858–862.

CHAPTER 4

1. Manufacturer's information: Viagra (Pfizer Inc., New York, NY); Levitra (GlaxoSmithKline, Brentford, Middlesex, UK); Cialis (Eli Lilly, Indianapolis, IN).
2. Porst H. Transurethral alprostadil with MUSE (medicated urethral system for erection) vs intracavernous alprostadil—a comparative study in 103 patients with erectile dysfunction. *Int J Impot Res* 1997; 9: 187–192.
3. Fulgham PF, Cochran JS, Denman JL, Feagins BA, Gross MB, Kadesky KT, et al. Disappointing initial results with transurethral alprostadil for erectile dysfunction in a urology practice setting. *J Urol* 1998; 160: 2041–2046.

CHAPTER 5

1. Sanda et al., *New Engl J Med* 2008; 358: 1250–1261.
2. Sanda et al., *New Engl J Med* 2008; 358: 1250–1261.
3. Blaivas JG, Marks BK, Weiss JP, Panagopoulos G & Somaroo C. Differential diagnosis of overactive bladder in men. *J Urol* 2009; 182: 2814–2818.
4. Sanda et al. *New Engl J Med* 2008; 358: 1250–1261.
5. Penson DF, McLerran D, Feng Z, Albertsen PC, Gilliland FD, Hamilton A, et al. 5-year urinary and sexual outcomes after radical prostatectomy: results from the prostate cancer outcomes study. *J Urol* 2005; 173: 1701–1705.
6. Kundu et al. *J Urol* 2004; 172: 2227–2231.

CHAPTER 6

1. Manassero F, Traversi C, Ales V, Pistolesi D, Panicucci E, Valent F, et al. Contribution of early intensive prolonged pelvic floor exercises on urinary continence recovery after bladder neck-sparing radical prostatectomy: results of a prospective controlled randomized trial., *Neurology and Urodynamics* 2007; 26: 985–989.

2. MacDonald R, Fink HA, Huckabay C, Monga M, & Wilt TJ. Pelvic floor muscle training to improve urinary incontinence after radical prostatectomy: a systematic review of effectiveness. *BJU Int* 2007; 100: 76–81.

3. Sacco E, Prayer-Galetti T, Pinto F, Fracalanza S, Betto G, Pagano F, et al. Urinary incontinence after radical prostatectomy: incidence by definition, risk factors and temporal trend in a large series with a long-term follow-up. *BJU Int* 2006; 97(6): 1234–1241.

4. Hay-Smith J, Herbison P, Ellis G, & Moore K. Anticholinergic drugs versus placebo for overactive bladder syndrome in adults. *Cochrane Database Syst Rev* 2002;(3): CD003781.

5. Schwinn DA & Roehrborn CG. Alpha1-adrenoceptor subtypes and lower urinary tract symptoms. *Int J Urol* 2008; 15(3): 193–199.

6. Lightner D, Calvosa C, Andersen R, Klimberg I, Brito CG, Snyder J, et al. A new injectable bulking agent for treatment of stress urinary incontinence: results of a multicenter,randomized, controlled, double-blind study of Durasphere. *Urology* 2001; 58(1):12–15.

7. Smith DN, Appell RA, Rackley RR, & Winters JC. Collagen injection therapy for post-prostatectomy incontinence. *J Urol* 1998; 160(2): 364–367.

8. Cornu JN, Sebe P, Ciofu C, Peyrat L, Beley S, Tligui M, et al. The AdVance Transobturator Male Sling for Post Prostatectomy Incontinence: Clinical results of a prospective evaluation after a minimum follow-up of 6 Months. *Eur Urol* 2009 56(6): 923–927.

9. Bauer RM, Bastian PJ, Gozzi C, & Stief CG. Postprostatectomy incontinence: all about diagnosis and management. *Eur Urol* 2009; 55(2): 322–333.

10. Gill BC, Swartz MA, Klein JB, Rackley RR, Montague DK, Vasavada SP, et al. Patient perceived effectiveness of a new male sling as treatment for post-prostatectomy incontinence. *J Urol* 2010; 183(1): 247–252.

11. Guimaraes M, Oliveira R, Pinto R, Soares A, Maia E, Botelho F, et al. Intermediate-term results, up to 4 years, of a bone-anchored male perineal sling for treating male stress urinary incontinence after prostate surgery. *BJU Int* 2009; 103(4): 500–504.

12. O'Connor, Lyon MB, Guralnick ML, & Bales GT. Long-term follow-up of single versus double cuff artificial urinary sphincter insertion for the treatment of severe postprostatectomy stress urinary incontinence. *Urology* 2008; 71(1): 90–93.

13. Hussain M, Greenwell TJ, Venn SN, & Mundy AR. The current role of the artificial urinary sphincter for the treatment of urinary incontinence. *J Urol* 2005; 174(2): 418–424.

14. Fulford SC, Sutton C, Bales G, Hickling M, & Stephenson TP. The fate of the 'modern' artificial urinary sphincter with a follow-up of more than 10 years. *Br J Urol* 1997; 79(5):713–716.

15. Kumar A, Litt ER, Ballert KN, & Nitti VW. Artificial urinary sphincter versus male sling for post-prostatectomy incontinence–what do patients choose? *J Urol* 2009; 181:1231–1235.

CHAPTER 7

1. Pal RP, Bhatt JR, Khan MA, Duggleby S, Camilleri P, Bell CR, et al. Prostatic length predicts functional outcomes after iodine-125 prostate brachytherapy. *Brachytherapy* 2010 doi:10.1016/j.brachy.2010.06.010.

2. Mabjeesh NJ, Chen J, Stenger A, & Matzkin H. Preimplant predictive factors of urinary retention after iodine 125 prostate brachytherapy. *Urology* 2007; 70(3): 548–553.

3. Mabjeesh et al. *Urology* 2007; 70(3): 548–553.

4. Cho KH, Lee CK, & Levitt SH. Proctitis after conventional external radiation therapy for prostate cancer: importance of minimizing posterior rectal dose. *Radiology* 1995; 195(3): 699–703.

5. Phan J, Swanson DA, Levy LB, Kudchadker RJ, Bruno TL, & Frank SJ. Late rectal complications after prostate brachytherapy for localized prostate cancer: incidence and management. *Cancer* 2009; 115(9): 1827–1839.

6. Lesperance RN, Kjorstadt RJ, Halligan JB, & Steele SR. Colorectal complications of external beam radiation versus brachytherapy for prostate cancer. *Am J Surg* 2008; 195(5):616–620.

7. Phan et al. *Cancer* 2009; 115(9): 1827–1839.

8. Lesperance et al. *Am J Surg* 2008; 195(5): 616–620.

9. Phan et al. *Cancer* 2009; 115(9): 1827–1839.

CHAPTER 8

1. Jemal et al. *CA Cancer J Clin* 2010;60(5): 277–300.

2. Armstrong AJ, Tannock IF, de Wit R, George DJ, Eisenberger M, & Halabi S. The development of risk groups in men with metastatic castration-resistant prostate cancer based on risk factors for PSA decline and survival. *Eur J Cancer* 2010; 46(3): 517–525.

3. Pound CR, Partin AW, Eisenberger MA, Chan DW, Pearson JD, & Walsh PC. Natural history of progression after PSA elevation following radical prostatectomy. *JAMA* 1999; 281: 1591–1597.

4. Bolla M, van Poppel H, Collette L, Van Cangh P, Vekemans K, Da Pozzo L, et al. Postoperative radiotherapy after radical prostatectomy: a randomised controlled trial (EORTC trial 22911). *Lancet* 2005; 366(9485): 572–578.

5. Thompson IM, Tangen CM, Paradelo J, Lucia MS, Miller G, Troyer D, et al. Adjuvant radiotherapy for pathological T3N0M0 prostate cancer significantly reduces risk of metastases and improves survival: long-term followup of a randomized clinical trial. *J Urol* 2009; 181: 956–962.

6. Wiegel T, Bottke D, Steiner U, Siegmann A, Golz R, Storkel S, et al. Phase III postoperative adjuvant radiotherapy after radical prostatectomy compared with radical prostatectomy alone in pT3 prostate cancer with postoperative undetectable prostate-specific antigen: ARO 96–02/AUO AP 09/95. *J Clin Oncol* 2009; 27: 2924–2930.

7. Thompson et al. *J Urol* 2009; 181(3): 956–962.

8. Wiegel T, Lohm G, Bottke D, Hocht S, Miller K, Siegmann A, et al. Achieving an undetectable PSA after radiotherapy for biochemical progression after radical prostatectomy is an independent predictor of biochemical outcome—results of a retrospective study. *Int J Radiat Oncol Biol Phys* 2009; 73(4): 1009–1016.

9. Wiegel et al. *Int J Radiat Oncol Biol Phys* 2009; 73: 1009–1016.

10. Bottke D, de Reijke TM, Bartkowiak D, & Wiegel T. Salvage radiotherapy in patients with persisting/rising PSA after radical prostatectomy for prostate cancer. *Eur J Cancer* 2009; 45 (Suppl 1): 148–157.

11. Wiegel et al. *Int J Radiation Oncology Biol Phys* 2009; 73: 1009–1016.

12. Huggins C & Hodges CV. Studies on prostate cancer 1. the effect of estrogen and of androgen injection on serum phosphatases in metastatic carcinoma of the prostate. *Cancer Res* 1941; 1: 293–297.

13. Bolla M, de Reijke TM, Van Tienhoven G, Van den Bergh AC, Oddens J, Poortmans PM, et al. Duration of androgen suppression in the treatment of prostate cancer. *N Engl J Med* 2009; 360(24): 2516–2527.

14. Iversen P, Tyrrell CJ, Kaisary AV, Anderson JB, Van Poppel H, Tammela TL, et al. Bicalutamide monotherapy compared with castration in patients with nonmetastatic locally advanced prostate cancer: 6.3 years of followup. *J Urol* 2000; 164(5): 1579–1582.

15. Mohile SG, Lacy M, Rodin M, Bylow K, Dale W, Meager MR, et al. Cognitive effects of androgen deprivation therapy in an older cohort of men with prostate cancer. *Crit Rev Oncol Hematol* 2010; 75(2): 152–159.

16. Morote J, Morin JP, Orsola A, Abascal JM, Salvador C, Trilla E, et al. Prevalence of osteoporosis during long-term androgen deprivation therapy in patients with prostate cancer. *Urology* 2007; 69(3): 500–504.

17. Smith MR. Bisphosphonates to prevent osteoporosis in men receiving androgen deprivation therapy for prostate cancer. *Drugs & Aging* 2003; 20(3): 175–183. And: Smith MR. Diagnosis and management of treatment-related osteoporosis in men with prostate carcinoma. *Cancer* 2003; 97(3 Suppl): 789–795.

18. Mohile SG, Mustian K, Bylow K, Hall W & Dale W Management of complications of androgen deprivation therapy in the older man. *Crit Rev Oncol Hematol* 2009; 70(3): 235–255.

19. Strum SB, McDermed JE, Scholz MC, Johnson H, & Tisman G. Anaemia associated with androgen deprivation in patients with prostate cancer receiving combined hormone blockade. *Br J Urol* 1997; 79(6): 933–941.

20. Messing, EM, Manola J, Sarosdy M, Wilding G, Crawford ED, & Trump D. Immediate hormonal therapy compared with observation after radical prostatectomy and pelvix lymphadenectomy in men with node-positive prostate cancer. *N Engl J Med* 1999; 341 (24): 1781–1788.

21. Bolla M, Gonzalez D, Warde P, Dubois JB, Mirimanoff RO, Storme G, et al. Improved survival in patients with locally advanced prostate cancer treated with radiotherapy and goserelin. *N Engl J Med* 1997; 337(5): 295–300.

CHAPTER 9

1. Bloch S, Love A, Macvean M, Duchesne G, Couper J & Kissane D. Psychological adjustment of men with prostate cancer: a review of the literature. *BioPsychoSocial Medicine* 2007; 10; 1: 2.

2. Kunkel EJ, Bakker JR, Myers RE, Oyesanmi O, Gomella LG. Biopsychosocial aspects of prostate cancer. *Psychosomatics* 2000; 41(2): 85–94.
3. Roth AJ. Improving quality of life: psychiatric aspects of treating prostate cancer, Psychiatric Times 2005; 22 Available at: psychiatrictimes.com/showArticle.jhtml?articleId=163101855 (Accessed 2/3/11).
4. Bloch et al. *BioPsychoSocial Medicine* 2007; 10; 1: 2.
5. Roth et al. *Psychiatric Times* 2005; 22.
6. Pirl WF & Mello J. Psychological complications of prostate cancer. *Oncology* (Williston Park). 2002; 16 (11): 1448–1453; discussion 1453–1454, 1457–1458, 1467.
7. Bloch et al. *BioPsychoSocial Medicine* 2007; 10; 1: 2.
8. Bloch et al. *BioPsychoSocial Medicine* 2007; 10; 1: 2.
9. Roth. *Psychiatric Times* 2005; 22.
10. Bloch et al. *BioPsychoSocial Medicine* 2007; 10: 1: 2.
11. Bloch et al. *BioPsychoSocial Medicine* 2007; 10: 1: 2.

CHAPTER 10

1. Soloway CT, Soloway MS, Kim SS, & Kava BR. Sexual, psychological and dyadic qualities of the prostate cancer 'couple.' *BJU International* 2005; 95(6): 780–785.
2. Matthew AG, Goldman A, Trachtenberg J, Robinson J, Horsburgh S, Currie K, et al. Sexual dysfunction after radical prostatectomy: prevalence, treatments, restricted use of treatments and distress. *J Urol* 2005; 174(6): 2105–2110.
3. Wittmann D, Northouse L, Foley S, Gilbert S, Wood DP Jr, Balon R, & Montie JE. The psychosocial aspects of sexual recovery after prostate cancer treatment, *Int J Impotence Res* 2009; 21: 99–106.
4. Monturo CA, Rogers PD, Coleman M, Robinson JP, Pickett M. Beyond sexual assessment: lessons learned from couples post radical prostatectomy. *J Am Acad Nurse Pract* 2001; 13 (11): 511–516.
5. Soloway et al. *BJU International*, 2005; 95(6): 780–785.
6. Soloway et al. *BJU International*, 2005; 95(6): 780–785.
7. Lepore SJ. A social-cognitive processing model of emotional adjustment to cancer. In: Baum A, Anderson B, editors. *Psychosocial Interventions for Cancer*. APA; Washington, DC: 2001. pp. 99–118.
8. Stanton AL, Danoff-Burg S, Cameron CL, Bishop M, Collins CA, Kirk SB, et al. Emotionally expressive coping predicts psychological and physical adjustment to breast cancer. *J Consult Clin Psychol* 2000; 68(5): 875–882.
9. Beck AM, Robinson JW, & Carlson LE. Sexual intimacy in heterosexual couples after prostate cancer treatment: what we know and what we still need to learn. *Urologic Oncology: Seminars and Original Investigations* 2009; 27: 137–143.
10. Wittmann et al. *Int J Impot Res* 2009; 21(2): 99–106.
11. Schover Leslie, telephone interview with R. Newnham, November 11, 2009.
12. Wittman et al. *Int J Impot Res.* 2009; 21(2): 99–106.
13. Monturo et al. *J Am Acad Nurse Pract* 2001; 13 (11): 511–516.
14. Soloway et al., *BJU International*, 2005; 95(6): 780–785.
15. Soloway et al. *BJU International*, 2005; 95(6): 780–785.

CHAPTER 11

1. Ahmed HU, Zacharakis E, Dudderidge T, Armitage JN, Scott R, Calleary J, et al. High-intensity-focused ultrasound in the treatment of primary prostate cancer: the first UK series. *Br J Cancer* 2009; 101(1): 19–26.

2. Eggener S, Gonzalgo M, & Yossepowitch O. Regarding: 'High-intensity-focused ultrasound in the treatment of primary prostate cancer: the first UK series'. *Br J Cancer* 2009; 101(12): 2057–2058.

3. Ripert T, Azémar MD, Ménard J, Bayoud Y, Messaoudi R, Duval F, et al. Transrectal high-intensity focused ultrasound (HIFU) treatment of localized prostate cancer: review of technical incidents and morbidity after 5 years of use. *Prostate Cancer Prostatic Dis* 2010; 13(2): 132–137.

4. Hoffmann NE & Bischof JC. The cryobiology of cryosurgical injury. *Urology* 2002; 60: 40–49.

5. Patel H, Mick R, Finlay J, Zhu TC, Rickter E, Cengel KA, et al. Motexafin lutetium-photodynamic therapy of prostate cancer: short- and long-term effects on prostate-specific antigen. *Clin Cancer Res* 2008; 14(15): 4869–4876.

6. Bivalacqua TJ, Deng W, Kendirci M, Usta MF, Robinson C, Taylor BK et al. Mesenchymal stem cells alone or ex vivo gene modified with endothelial nitric oxide synthase reverse age-associated erectile dysfunction. *Am J Physiol Heart Circ Physiol* 2007; 292(3): H1278–H1290.

7. Kato R., Wolfe D, Coyle CH, Wechuck JB, Tyagi P, Tsukamoto T, et al. Herpes simplex virus vector-mediated delivery of neurturin rescues erectile dysfunction of cavernous nerve injury. *Gene Ther* 2009; 16(1); 26–33.

8. Smaldone MC. & Chancellor MB. Muscle derived stem cell therapy for stress urinary incontinence. *World J Urol* 2008; 26(4): 327–332.

9. Smaldone MC, Chen ML, & Chancellor MB. Stem cell therapy for urethral sphincter regeneration. *Minerva Urol Nefrol* 2009; 61(1): 27–40.

10. Tedesco FS, Dellavalle A, Diaz-Manera J, Messina G, Cossu G. Repairing skeletal muscle: regenerative potential of skeletal muscle stem cells. *J Clin Invest* 2010; 120(1): 11–19.

11. Kato et al. *Gene Ther* 2009; 16(1): 26–33.

12. Strasser H, Berjukow S, Marksteiner R, Margreiter E, Hering S, Bartsch G et al. Stem cell therapy for urinary stress incontinence. *Exp Gerontol* 2004; 39(9): 1259–1265.

13. Kato et al. *Gene Ther* 2009; 16(1): 26–33.

14. Mitterberger M, Marksteiner R, Margreiter E, Pinggera GM, Frauscher F, Ulmer H et al. Myoblast and fibroblast therapy for post-prostatectomy urinary incontinence: 1-year followup of 63 patients. *J Urol* 2008; 179(1): 226–231.

15. Abbott A, Doctors accused of doing illegal stem-cell trials; patients in Austria may have been misled. *Nature* 2008; 453(7191): 6–7.

16. Strasser H. Stem-cell urological treatment was not carried out illegally. *Nature* 2008; 453(7199): 1177.

17. Melman A, Bar-Chama N, McCullough A, Davies K & Christ G. The first human trial for gene transfer therapy for the treatment of erectile dysfunction: preliminary results. *Eur Urol* 2005; 48(2): 314–318.

18. Melman A, Bar-Chama N, McCullough A, Davies K, Christ G. hMaxi-K gene transfer in males with erectile dysfunction: results of the first human trial. *Hum Gene Ther* 2006; 17(12): 1165–1176.

19. Bivalacqua TJ, Deng W, Champion HC, Hellstrom WJ, & Kadowitz PJ. Gene therapy techniques for the delivery of endothelial nitric oxide synthase to the corpora cavernosa for erectile dysfunction. *Methods Mol Biol* 2004; 279: 173–185.

20. Bivalacqua et al, *Am J Physiol Heart Circ Physiol* 2007; 292(3): H1278–H1290.

21. Kato et al, *Gene Ther* 2009; 16(1): 26–33.

ABOUT THE AUTHORS

ARNOLD MELMAN, MD, is Professor and Chairman of the Department of Urology at the Albert Einstein College of Medicine/Montefiore Medical Center.

ROSEMARY E. NEWNHAM is the former Assistant Director of the Oral History Research Office at Columbia University, where she earned her MFA in nonfiction writing. She works with Columbia's Narrative Medicine program and is a medical writer.